Claudio Ronco

–THE CONNECTIVIST–

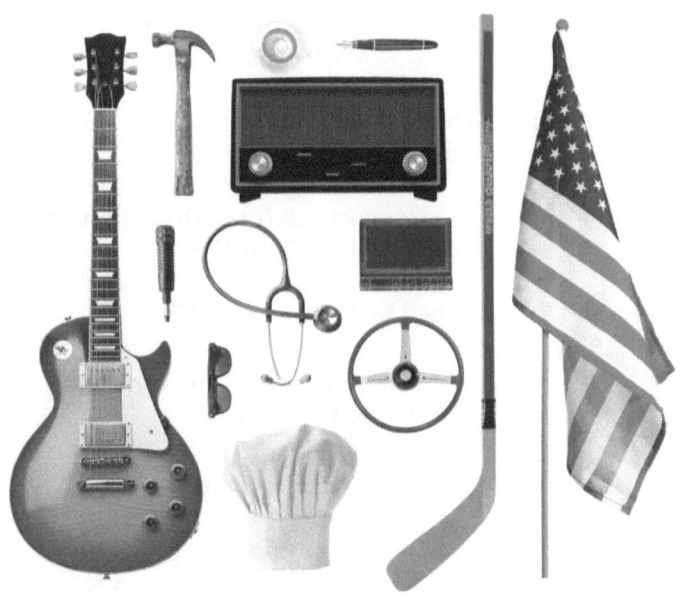

Copyright 2022 by the author Claudio Ronco, M.D.

The book author retains sole copyright to his contributions to this book.

All rights reserved. No portion of this book may be reproduced, stored in a retrieval system, or transmitted in any form or by any means — electronic, mechanical, photocopy, recording, scanning, or other — except for brief quotations in critical reviews or articles, without the prior written permission of the author.

Published 2022. Printed in the United States of America and distributed Internationally by Ingram Group.

1st Edition - 2016, Il Connettivista (Italian) Perfect Paperback
ISBN-13: 978-88-942722-4-6

2nd Edition - 2020, The Connectivist (English) Perfect Paperback
ISBN 978-1-950647-59-0

2nd Edition - 2022, The Connectivist (English) Perfect Paperback
ISBN 978-1-957077-04-8

Published by Fondazione IRRIV.

English translation: MaryLou Wratten, Gioia Vencato

Cover art: Michele Zorzetto

Book layout and formatting by:
BookCrafters, Parker, Colorado, USA
http://bookcrafters.net

Definition of Connectivism: A learning theory that recognizes the evolution of ever-changing learning networks, their complexity, and the role that technology plays in learning networks through facilitation of existing learning networks and creation of new learning networks.

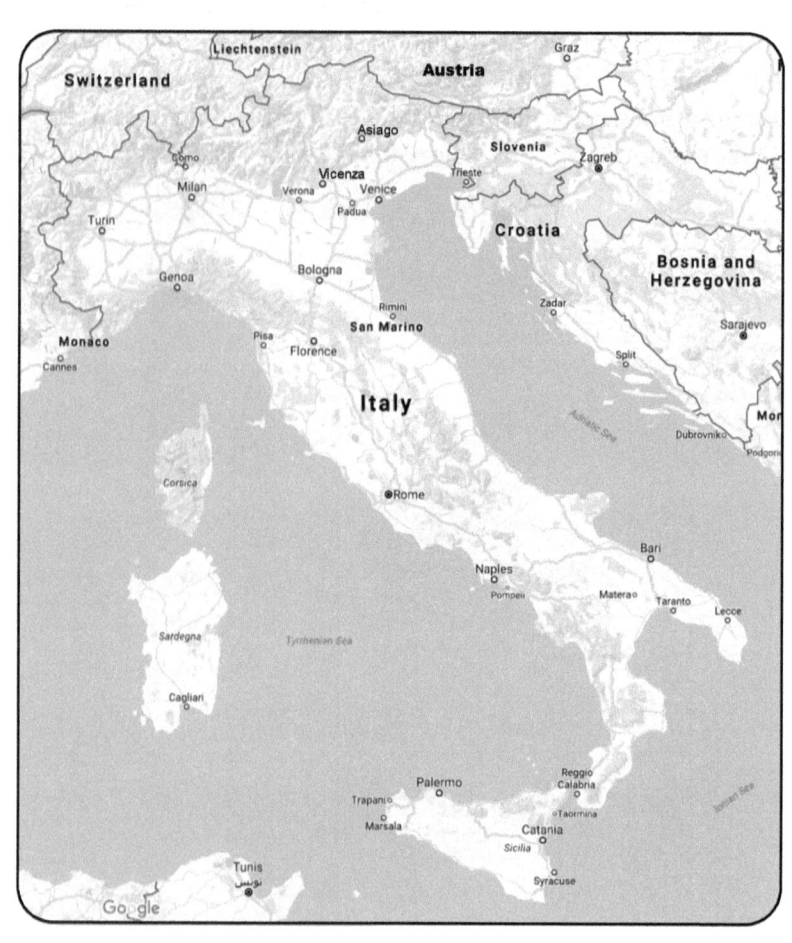

Table of Contents

From within the darkness of illness to the light of passion 1

Prologue 3

  I. The age of play 5
      The Peter Pan Syndrome 7
      To Study and learn 16
      Eloquence by example 19
  II. The game of life 23
      Doctor like my father 25
      Lifestyle 29
      The American dream 32
      Language and use 40
      Giulietta, the passion of a lifetime 44
  III. Time for Responsibility 55
      The connectivist 57
      Ethics and the art of being cured 63
      The Water of life 72
      Navigating into profound space 81
      Carpediem 88
      The story of Gio' — born and born again ... 95
      Cooking healthy food for the kidneys 117

IV.	From the past to the future............................	123
	Teachers and mentors.................................	125
	Irrivians forever!..	129
	Gaudeamus igitur.......................................	135
V.	Live life to the fullest...................................	141
	Note from the heart....................................	143
	The magic of ice...	154
	Festina lente (Hurry Slowly).......................	164
	Shangri-La...	173

***Epilogue*... 181**

***About the Author*.. 183**

Dedication

To Paola, my partner of passion
To Federico, my partner of play
To Umberto, Light within the darkness of silliness
To my colleagues, my partners of learning
To my students, my partners of experience
To my friends, the real ones
To my parents, who will always live within me
And to Giancarlo, great man of principle
and infinite generosity

From within the darkness of illness to the light of passion

THE INSPIRATION FOR THIS BOOK was largely due to Umberto Veronesi, the scientist that completely changed the way to approach women's breast cancer and, through his research, saved thousands of lives. Prof Veronesi was the creator and director of the Istituto Internazionale per la Cura dei Tumori (International Institute for the Cure of Tumors). He was a model as a physician, research scientist and over the last years, a dear friend.

I met him in person when I invited him to come to Vicenza to the inauguration of our Istituto Internazionale di Ricerca Renale (International Institute of Renal Research) with the discovery of many things in common between his specialty of Oncology and ours of Nephrology. I was really pleased that his mentorship was shared within our group stating that the sick patient should always be at the forefront of a physician's life and that medicine cannot exist without culture. Medicine isn't a pure science like mathematics or philosophy. It rather responds to the necessity of the sick patient as a person and it should always match with high ethical standards to be correct.

Our friendship was further strengthened when he agreed to write the preface to my first book, *Carpediem*, the story of a baby girl that was saved by the creation of a dedicated miniaturized machine for pediatric dialysis. That machine was the result of a perseverant research of a physician able to materialize his dreams unifying the formal structure of patient care with the didactic nature of research.

I couldn't have hoped for a better introduction to that book, which should have been my first and last writing experience. On the contrary, on the occasion of our last meeting in Milan a few weeks before he passed away, he stimulated me to put in writing my experiences and my passions. His words have left with me a profound message. "Dear Claudio,"- he whispered — "let your experience and your passions flow within and tell others about yourself trying to understand more about who you are. I see inside you things that you may not even imagine and that will emerge from your writings. Move fast from the painful experiences of your medical profession to the light and joyful moments of your life. Move from the darkness of illness to the light of passion. Keep writing for yourself, for your friends, for your patients, because we all need to live our dreams and follow our passions."

In this second book, the one that you are reading now, I tried to extract my internal emotions and to describe them through a series of episodes in which passion and love are the common denominator. I tried to recount the passion and dreams of a young physician and researcher though a story of illness and recovery of mind and body, the Story of Gio', that in a certain sense, continues to complete the journey started in *Carpediem*.

It is a book for the young fellow and the mature person. It is a book full of emotions that takes the reader through the imagination and the dreams of someone with the experience of a full university professor and the soul of Peter Pan.

Prologue

PATRAS, 20 SEPTEMBER 2017. The ceremony has concluded the welcome address and preliminary openings, but in my mind I keep going back to the recent charity rock concert where we performed in front of 900 people with songs from the 70s to finance the research activities for the Istituto di Ricerca Renale di Vicenza (IRRIV). Tomorrow I will depart for my annual series of conferences at the University of New York, for which the American Society of Nephrology has dedicated an entire week in the Big Apple. But today, I am at the oldest University in Greece, the school of Esculapio — father of modern medicine, to receive my honorary degree.

They dress me in the traditional robes of the university and give me the necklace with the cross of Patras, the symbol of their teaching doctrine. I begin my keynote lecture, incorporating philosophy, applied science, engineering, biology, medicine and even including elements of modern nanotechnology linking everything with the theories of Galileo. It is in fact, the content of my life as a physician-scientist that brought me to invent Carpediem, the machine that saved so many neonates from the insidious disease of acute renal failure. I have one hour of slides and data that are sprinkled with anecdotes and passionate stories about my life — the patients, research, teaching budding young professionals, ice hockey, cooking, music, writing, vintage cars, sailing, and my mounts. At the end of the speech from the dean — a professor of philosophy, he gives me a warm academic hug and turns to the public declaring with a friendly joke that the title of the degree that I was given, honoris causa was actually a duplicate in both medicine and humanities. He then turns to me and asks "…but how do you do all of these things together Professor? You must have very little time for sleeping!"

I replied "Actually, I can hardly get out of bed in the morning and I am also a little lazy. At home, I was the slowest in the family and for all my life I had to run to demonstrate that I wasn't below the others. As such, I learned by experience to do things like opening Windows on my computer: I open many windows simultaneously and try and manage them to my best all at once. I also admit that if I don't get enough sleep. I have great difficulty performing at my best. I am like a laptop with the batteries at zero — even if there is a superfast processor. Fortunately, I am able to sleep on command and utilize short naps of ten minutes or one hour depending on the available time. I turn myself off for a little, just like the robot C3PO in *Star Wars*."

Everyone laughs and applauds, but my thoughts are already on the entrance to the conference hall at Columbia University. In the same manner, when I am physically giving lessons in New York, my mind wanders to being aboard the sailboat of my friend Mauro where I will rest before flying to Peking for the Chinese Society of Nephrology congress. Just as the saying goes, men who stop are lost. From my first trip to New York in 1982 to today, I think I have traveled around the world at least a hundred times. From East to West, and vice versa, in a continuous spiral of time zones, jet lag, language, different cultures, lifestyles and regulations. This was not done for pleasure, but rather with great pleasure. So, you might ask, how do you arrive at this frenetic way of life. It is a strange story, but ordinary and at the same time extraordinary, well-planned but often irrational, and at the origin, there is perhaps the Peter Pan Syndrome.

I. The age of play

«È dentro noi un fanciullino che ha brividi, lacrime e tripudi suoi»

"It is inside us a child that has emotions, tears and joy."

—*Giovanni Pascoli*

The Peter Pan Syndrome

THERE ARE THOSE who never grow up, and those who never want to grow up. In reality, the ideal situation would be to mix these two realities in adolescence: maturity and old age with just the right dose of the irrationality and spontaneity of a child. The child that lives deep within us has a desire to exit and discover, live and experience joy. Some of us suppress this inner child, while others let the child have free rein. This leads to some people as appearing positively infantile and enthusiastic for life, while other appear (at least apparently) mature, but often with an aura of sadness.

One-time John Lennon was asked the question of what he wanted to be when he grew up and he replied, "to be happy." When some object and say that maybe he didn't understand the question, he replied that certainly they didn't understand life.

I have always felt as though there was always a childlike presence; from my infancy, to childhood and maybe also now that I am living in the last part of my life. There have always been people that have tried to suggest that my character contained a little too much of the childlike nature. I don't agree. Instead, I am just not embarrassed and think it is fine to let this child shine in the moments of my life. I believe that this has probably saved me from having a nervous breakdown or depression and maintained my life in a positive and active manner.

If it is true that most people hide their inner child, there are some individuals that expose this child with great pride. I remember a conversation with the poet and language historian, Fernando Bandini. One night in May, at the Accademia Olimpica di Vicenza (Olympic Academy in Vicenza), in which he was president, we had a conference on nanotechnology and medicine, a theme which potentially could be considered as dangerously boring. Fernando instead said that my speech made him think of an episode from the television series *Star Trek*, in which little self-replicated robots had taken over the Starship Enterprise. He continued to tell the story of the episode where it had been suggested to the producer from the writings of Eric Drexler, the father of nanotechnology, in which the discovery of a new discipline had been born more from creative fantasy of certain individuals with personalities and nature almost as philosophers rather than mere "scientists." At that point, the poet and philologist couldn't resist the temptation to share with me that his favorite evening reading was from the comic books from Tex Willer and continued to tell me about the various episodes mixing social theories sprinkled with philosophical citations that made me understand at that moment, that only if you think like a child, that you will allow your mind to be open to innovation. That night we continued to discuss this point at length.

There are different types of innovation. Incremental innovation and radical innovation. Incremental innovations are the inventions that occur in small steps and allow us to move forward in a slow determined manner. These are often the work of groups of organized small or even large groups and often make up entire departments of "Research and Development." These incremental inventions are important for making things more useful, but not sufficient to change the world. The radical innovations, however, are events that are the incredible gift from minds free of boundaries, with benefits that can disrupt and change the world. They can push and provoke quantum leaps that allow humanity to enter phases of a new story.

Interestingly, the term 'quantum' derives from particle

physics, where levels of energy exist and we can differentiate orbital electrons from those that are internal to an atom. This isn't a continuum, but rather a true and real state with differences between one level and another, in much the same way that a switch can be turned on or off. Examples of radical innovation include the discovery of penicillin, radio waves and motors. The internal combustion engine was an invention that profoundly changed the world. In a short time, the technology was nearly brought to perfection, but to achieve this — to make a quantum leap — both the motor and the reaction to the technology, were needed. This is also what helped us break the sound barrier and even reach the moon.

In science fiction books, even inexperienced readers know that sooner or later there will be challenge on how to reach the stars. The distance in light years between the earth and nearby stars makes it impossible to reach the stars with help from our actual motors. We will need propulsion engines that still haven't been invented. The problem will resolve when someone that doesn't realize that the problem seems impossible and looks at it with childlike curiosity and ingenuity to resolve and invent a new "star motor." The mind of a child — or even the fractional percentage of the child's mind that still exists within us, is the essential ingredient for any type of radical innovation. If you try and ask a child to solve a complex problem, or even a young student sheltered from the current scientific approach to the problem, you will be amazed at the ideas that can arise. Never underestimate the ideas of a child, and even more so the ideas of a passionate reader of science fiction.

The child that is within all of us as adults, is the same one as in infancy. With time, ideas and thought are structured differently, but the intrinsic nature of the child within us remains. Our memories also remain. These are not simple fragments of DNA stored and warehoused within our brain, but rather constitute the imprinting we hold for our entire life.

***

My first years at school, followed by those of elementary school and middle school were fantastic in that they were simple, serene and full of happiness. The altitude of 1000 meters and the nature of the Altopiano di Asiago (Asiago region), made the landscape come alive each month due to temperature and seasonal changes that gave the opportunity to play in an ever-changing landscape. We had intense cold in January and February, in which we had great fun in the snow and on the ice. The youngest remained close to home building snowmen and small igloos while the older children had snowball fights or sledding on a simple piece of cardboard. Those that had wooden skis or reinforced sleds could descend with great velocity on the trail of "Seven heads" or the "Parco di rimembranza" or San Domenico. At the last days of Carnivale, the toys were transferred to the masked wagons prepared by the different districts. My brothers went in masks (made very economically) by Aunt Rita and Aunt Ninetta. For the classic Pierrot, all that was needed was a white jumpsuit with three or four big black buttons. I didn't like wearing a mask though and preferred to be the Harlequin, cheerful and playful. One year the Aunts returned from a trip from Spain, organized by the local congregation, and dressed us as bullfighters. We stayed on the balcony above the old pharmacy and practiced "skewering the bull," made from a cardboard head and an old cowhide, when the wagons passed by.

Spring always began with the tradition of " Shella Marzo." Boys would parade through the streets of the town with small cups and sheet metal to scare away the winter spirits with noise. This was followed by the burning of the vecia (old witch) with singing in the main square.

Schella, schella Marzo / snea dehin / gras dehear / alle de Dillen lear. // Az der Kucko kuck / pluut der balt. / Ber lange lebet / sterbet alt

(Sounds March / off the snow / here the grass / all the barns

empty. // When the cuckoo sings / flowers the forest. / Who lives a long time / dies old)

If the snow started to melt away early, we would play ball in any open space between he houses or in the churchyard. The steps of the churchyard would also serve as tracks for competitions with soda pop tops, while the girls would play scalon or prison ball (strange games that we, boys, could not understand). In April, the days would alternate between warm days and unexpected snowfall. This would frustrate our plans, as we were eager to resume our football matches that had been abandoned during the long winter months. Sometimes they would shovel the playground because it had already been decided that winter was finished and we just had to play at any cost. May was characterized by long afternoons with breathless runs in the courtyards. Children would scream and yell and this mixed pleasantly with the cheeps and chirps from the swallows. In the evenings, with the excuse of the "fioretto della Madonna," we would go out hunting for beetles. We would make them fly like helicopters while holding them with a wire tied to one leg.

Between the months of May and June, there was a large ancient religious procession, Grande Rogazione, that passed through an area of the Altopiano, that we treated like an adventure and game. In June, at the end of school we were free to fly kites and play big football matches. We made a type of local "summer Olympics" with relative handmade carved wooden medals. In July, if you were under 13, you went hunting for birds with a slingshot, while the older boys started the "hunt for girls" staying in the area on holiday. August was the month of the Prunno festival, a gathering not far from the town where a queen of the forest was chosen and typical games from the area consisted of sack races, ring tosses, breaking of the pignata and climbing the tree to get the goblet. The festival ended with a torchlight procession to the Millepini Park and fireworks. Summer practically ended on the first Sunday after August 15 when the tourists started to return home to the cities or outlying suburbs and the local boys were again masters of the area.

In Autumn, the woods were blanketed by beautiful colors with splashes of red from the beech trees and orange from the larch trees. Then, towards the first days of October, we began to notice the particular smell of smoke, wet wood, resin and the essential oils of pine that made up a type of natural diffusor with essences that warmed the heart. The beech stele (inner part of the bark) burned in inexpensive wood burning stoves and warmed the dining rooms. The games moved more frequently inside the house, in the corridors and in the rooms close to the stairs, and sometimes in an attic with creaky wooden floors or inside the patronato (charitable institution).

In November, around the festival remembering the dead, the first snow would begin to fall and the anxious stadium warden would decide whether or not to convert the stadium to with ice for Ice hockey. For months at home, we would wait for "real ice" after practicing in the hallways with broom handles and wooden tablets. In December, we lived the poetry of Christmas. We wandered through the woods gathering crib moss to sell from house to house. We used the earnings from the moss, together with the savings already collected from the sales of old iron and relics of the Great War (found in the fields) to make our team's football shirt. In the evenings we would go for the choir tests and to prepare the Missa Pontificalis of the priest Don Lorenzo Peronsi in order to prepare to sing on Christmas Eve.

Just as every season offered us games and different degrees of happiness in Asiago, it also stimulated and aroused our curiosity and wonder every day. Each child's eyes, are by nature, are wonderful because they reflect the ingenuity and purity of being human, but not being contaminated by the miseries of the world.

For me, everything was a source of amazement. To be able to witness a calf being born in the stable of Bepi on the

Contrada Busa, hear the Mattio, the bell of the cathedral, to play for the festival of the hay or the hammer bell sounding like a fire or misfortune. I marveled at the flags of the Alpini waving in the square, admired the floral compositions that were created by ice on the windows and watched with wonder at the baby robins hatching in their nests. We listened with as the winds screeched and crossed the forest and with anticipation to the stories from old people told while sitting next to the fireplace. We lived a simple life in the village: but filled with so many wonderful things. It really did give me joy. I was happy with whatever happened to me, it was as though it was the most beautiful and extraordinary thing that could have happened. I lived in the constant and feverish expectation that tomorrow would be a new day that would be reserved for me. Without really realizing it at the time, this helped me to develop my psychological attitude that would be the basis and my predilection and stimulus for research.

***

I dreamed of doing research ever since I was a child. I wasn't sure, at the time, where this would be but I was determined that this was what I wanted to do. I looked at the world around me. I looked at every fragment of life as under the microscope lens, and I realized that problems were everywhere. In ninety percent of the cases, I could find solutions using the laws of physics or biology explained in the *Treasury Encyclopedia* or just from the answers of Uncle Gigi, the family scientist that constantly produced many small inventions. I've learned since then an important thing: that to solve a problem you need to have the modesty to seek and seek since almost always someone has already thought of it. With our research and our solutions — we can only add a few solid bricks to the scientific "wall of science" and contribute to the final architecture of the building. Galileo used to say that in order to advance science, one must descend from the cornucopia of "the possible" and find a small piece that is able to be demonstrated. Together we can query the various networks to see if there is a problem that lacks certain answers and then proceed with prudence and modesty in a research project of our own. Although it will be the scientific method that will help to make it solid; the feasibility analysis that will help make it sustainable and the fair management of resources that will help us make it achievable, it is the enthusiasm from the heart of the child within us that will drive us forward.

It is not easy to start from a blank sheet of paper, design a device from nothing, enunciate a hypothesis to be tested with the scientific method. But it is the heart of the child we have inside that makes us exceed every rational obstacle and keep us going by seeing a possible result that other do not see. We can find random but extraordinary discoveries and the problems that arise before us are sometimes false problems.

Jules Verne was a good example of someone that moved with the heart of a child. For him, it wasn't important that needed to be brought to the man on the moon, but how to house the chickens that would provide fresh eggs on the way. In the movie *2001 Space Odyssey*, the HAL 9000 computer was a real one and an example of artificial intelligence, even if the screen worked still with green LEDs and primitive graphics. The multi-tasking was beyond coming but the seed of the calculator thinker had already been planted in the fertile field of science fiction that would soon become science.

The realities of this issue create endless problems. Federico Faggin, the inventor of the microchip told me that we will never have a truly aware and conscious computer, and that maybe even the computer would need an irrational child within its circuits, but this at most will always be the result of an interventional planned by the creator. The future is open. It is just a matter of time and those who can see beyond the present will not only imagine the world of the future, but will also help create it.

Steve Jobs was famous for seeing beyond reality, and in many cases, his mind operated as a type of real distortion on realities. His intuition was like child's play. Only those who can think like a child will become successful at research, because all research is made up of attempts to succeed in something that seems impossible. After all, if the solution seemed possible, it would have already been found and there would be no need for a new project.

To study and learn

STUDY AND LEARN. Learn and study. This is the greatest wealth that one can accumulate. This was repeated to me over and over by my parents. In junior high, I had everything in mind BUT to study, and since my mother was the daughter of a carabiniere (policeman), I couldn't avoid doing homework under her supervision. And yet despite this, one year I still succeeded in having my transition to the next year put "on hold." Our professor of Italian, Latin, history and geography was also the mayor of the town and was therefore constantly called out of the classroom to sign documents and attend to his other duties. This allowed us the opportunity to find questions prepared for our homework. As a result, we didn't learn very much that year and in the third year of junior high school I failed my exam in history and geography. I ended up studying the entire summer from the course of the Danube, the countries of the Baltic sea and the l'epopea (epic) of Carlo Magno and the Habsburg instead of going out with Christina, a girl of brown hair and big fawn eyes. Since I always hated history, I learned geography studying the thousands of routes of aircraft that I have used as an adult to fly around the world.

After passing the rocky middle school third year, I decided that I should take control of my own destiny and also address the problem of which collegio (high school boarding school) to choose for my further studies. In general, the students at the collegio were two types: those considered as inmates as punishment because they were refractory to studying or those that were considered as exiles from areas that lacked high schools. I was in the exile group — sad and a little disoriented. At fourteen, living away from home, in a somewhat hostile atmosphere wasn't easy. To gain the respect of the others, you needed to immediately cordon off your space and make it clear that you weren't weak. I gained that respect almost immediately after a series of conflicts — sometimes even violent, with the vice dean, a grim priest that weighed over a hundred kilos; the prefect, a university student that had free board and lodging, but that was in charge of the supervision of us, and with the custodian, a wiry man who always had a cigarette in his mouth and wouldn't let us use the volleyball court because we ruined the flower beds. In the eyes of my fellow students, one that quarreled with the system was in fact a man with earned respect. This meant I was able to choose the place at the table, enter first in the soccer room, leave my pen on the counter without risk that it would be taken and having the bed that was the farthest from the prefect (a university student that had free board and lodging) in the dormitory. Although these might seem like little things in the world of the collegio — they were very similar to that of the barracks and they counted. But I remained with a burning nostalgia for the Altopiano and my far away friends, that even weekend and long summer breaks couldn't extinguish.

As I grew older, I was still interested in games, but they became more serious and useful for the purposes of my training. Although I wasn't a model student, I always had a good dose of perseverance (sometimes referred to as stubbornness). From an early age, I thought that if someone had managed to do something, then I could do that too, as long as I had the right application and time. Maybe a little better, or a little worse, but I could have done it. Under my home was the workshop of a shoemaker. I would watch for hours as Attilio would adjust shoes or cut the skin to make the double uppers. He was an artist and there was much to learn. At the age of twelve, I changed my first pair of soles on my moccasins that I had worn out playing soccer. What satisfaction! Riccardo Girardini instead was a carpenter who made incastri a coda di rondine - dovetail wedges, like no one else. It took me a long time to convince him to let me use his tools and machines, because the workers needed to keep up with the work and there was no time to play. One year later however I spent the entire summer learning carpentry and at the end of August he let me paste, cut and mill. The father of my friend Flavio often sent us to mount antennas from customers who had just purchased a television. It wasn't an easy task because the signal was weak and one of us would have to stay on the roof, even for hours, before being able to adjust the tuning on the only channel that was transmitted by the state television station RAI. We also did other little odd jobs such as electricians or by offering to replace kitchen gas cylinders. That was how some of us learned a trade, while others practiced manual skills or acquired the ability to creatively solve problems and find practical solutions that would be useful in securing success in a future profession. This was true at least in my case, since the taste of invention and skill remained ingrained within me, even when I no longer had anything to do with shoe uppers or electric circuits, but rather as a nephrologist with circuits, blood vessels - tangles of vessels and thin catheters.

Eloquence by example

I STILL REMEMBER so many times as a boy seeing my father get up from the table in the middle of dinner, put on his coat, take his bag and disappear without understanding the reason. One day, when I was about five years old, I was out walking with my mother and we were stopped by a poorly dressed lady who carried a basket on her arm. She lifted the kitchen towel from the basket and offered us two eggs with a shy but friendly and heartfelt gesture. At that moment, the gesture was incomprehensible for me, but evidently not for my mother. Another time, more or less at the same age, I realized that my favorite blanket that had a border of Mickey Mouse and that I had called my catata had disappeared. At first, I didn't receive an answer to my question, but after much insistence, I was told that the blanket had been used in the delivery of a child. How in the world could a blanket give birth to a child!? I didn't understand the explanation, but I took it anyway. At the age of six, I went with my parents to Lazzaretto to attend the Grande Rogazione. The festival was THE event for the town, with the shops closed and everyone participating in the procession or at least the mass. On that occasion, women prepared baskets of boiled eggs colored with the juices of herbs and spring flowers to give to men as a sign of friendship, admiration, sympathy and gratitude for a favor or act of kindness. Among the many eggs we received, there was always one that was specially decorated: the one intended to the special person "of the heart." Considering that my father could of course not be considered as the preferred person of all the women from the village, but judging from the quantity of eggs that he received, I had to conclude that he had the deep gratitude and admiration of many. Also that day, my father had to leave early from his snack, since a boy had come running from the Asiago district saying in a breathless manner that his mother had fainted. I began to understand what it meant to be a general doctor of the town — not a doctor of many, but just being a doctor was enough. My father's character was seemed to be rather "gruff." When he got home, he didn't utter a word. He sat down at the table at exactly 1 p.m. for lunch and at 19:30 in the evening. He was precise to the minute. If I forgot to wash my hands, he would mumble grumpily. He wanted order and didn't appreciate noise. Silence at the table would put him in a good mood. Actually my father was an extraordinary man with an incredible humanity. I only noticed this with time, when I came to my own senses! Today, knowing the profession and the stories that a doctor is forced to live by sharing the suffering of his patients, I can understand the shadows that passed over his face in the evening and the thoughts that dwelled in his mind.

Have you ever wondered why everyone complains about the lack of the old family doctor? "Ah, how we had the greatest family doctor — it was enough to just look you in the eyes to make a diagnosis." Those were good times when the doctor would come to the house and we would prepare the clean towels for him to wash his hands after the visit with the grandmother who was sick in bed for a long time! The doctor would listen with patience to that stubborn Toni trying to make him understand that his daughter was old enough (and had the right) to get married. But where did the good family doctor go, the one that knew everything about grandparents, fathers and children and families as well as the town's problems? In reality, that doctor's life was far from easy. Despite the great gratitude and high esteem, the doctor's had horrific hours. They were on call 7 days a week,

24 hours a day. They had modest salaries and enormous responsibilities. In Italian, the term "medico condotto" was used to refer to a physician that was employed by the town, that gave service free of charge to those that couldn't pay and modest fees for others according to an established table. The term condotto (conduct in English) actually derives precisely from a directive from the post-war Ministry of the Interior that provided for the *medico condotto* to take residence in an area and take care of the poor and sick of that community. The mountain doctor had the further disadvantage of the unexpected and often challenging weather, that would make some missions even more complicated. My father would rely only on his inseparable bag and his trusty Topolino C, a little car, that disappeared one day in 1955 and reappeared a year later. I eventually found out that the mortgage repayments were not compatible with his medical doctor's salary.

The only moments that my brother and I could share with my father were those immediately after lunch, when, in the absence of urgent calls he would allow us to walk along the trails of the Great War. At that time, the Altopiano of Asiago was an open air museum and a naturalistic encyclopedia that he would patiently illustrate to us. We stopped in the clearings of the Castelloni of San Marco where we heard the call of the Capercaillie (grouse) when he would try and attract the attention of nearby females. We would remain hidden, to observe his love dance. Sometimes my father would take us towards the Porta Manazzo and the Portule to show us, in the Val Formica, the marmots coming out of their dens like the ship's watchmen and they would whistle to send themselves warning signs. We were walking along the heights of Kaberlaba in search of Morel mushrooms or after the disappearance of the last snow to the Mazze to collect daffodils for my mother. I can't tell if those memories are so alive and happy because my father was with me, or if I have an olfactory memory of the extraordinary moments of my life. They say that the sense of smell is the oldest of our senses which can bring us actually ancestral reminiscence. Not by chance, the sensory location is precisely in the archipallio (archipallio of the hippocampus), the phylogenetically oldest part of our brain. Of course ours tends to expand in a temporal manner during the most beautiful moments and contract during those that are more difficult.

One day I passed in front of a shop while going to school and the owner called me inside to give me some little statues and houses for the nativity crib. I had gone there the day before to buy a small papier-mache mill, that I had intended to add, just as in previous years with a new piece. I guess the shopkeeper had seen my indecision and the time I had taken to choose the piece and understood that I could not afford more than one. I think he thought this was a good opportunity to repay the doctor. As I realized only later, the lady had me filled with gifts, because my father had passed by their house every morning and evening to give an injection to her husband that suffered from an incurable disease. The benefit for the patient didn't depend only on the injection, but also the chat with my father and the coffee that they shared together. In fact, the coffee was the only thing that would remain in the stomach of the patient, while the rest of what he ate during the day was usually vomited up. The words of hope and the stories of the last trip to the mountains are what kept the man alive, and gave him the gift of hope that next season they would go to the woods together.

Another case, this time solved by my father with a "creative method," was that of a photographer who suffered from a very painful ulcer. For three months he added a solemn feast of polenta and salami or sauerkraut and cheese to our afternoon strolls. After this therapy "food shock," stress was defeated and the ulcer too! From then the postcards that the photographer produced were, in a manner of speaking, more alive and colorful and cheerful.

II. The game of life

"Drop your moorings, get out of the safe harbor
and let the wind blow your sail."

—*Mark Twain*

Doctor like my father

IN THE SUMMER OF 1968, a great meeting was held at my house to decide whether I could face the pitfalls and challenges of a sprawling city like Vicenza to attend a public high school. The decision was positive, and my parents rented a room for me near Ponte Pusterla. I found myself in the home of a nice older woman who hosted me for three years, acting as my aunt, mother and also grandmother. It was incredible. I could hardly believe that I passed from a dormitory of 50 beds from the college to a single room with my own bathroom. Finally, I was able to study alone, go in and out of the house when I wanted and even have lunch and dinners with food prepared to my own tastes. My school was located a few hundred meters from the house. It was the famous Liceo Pigafetta, known for its high quality and standards and the severity of the professors. But what really interested me was the fact that it was a mixed high school. Over half the students had skirts and long hair. Actually, in the year 1968, even some of the boys started wearing their hair longer, as the winds of change had been blowing for some time. California and France had demonstrations and choregraphed scenes where intense discussions of Sartre and Marcuse merged with those of Che's feats and the waving of Mao's red book in the processions of student groups. Feminists were engaged in the campaign for the bra-less liberation of the breasts. From my perspective though — I loved that moment in my life and didn't really feel the need for change.

I found the period carefree, happy and full of perfumes and emotions, even without having to resort to ideologic motivators, alcohol or use of drugs. Excitement provided me with enough hormones that were generating intoxicating moments of falling for a beloved conquest or phases of black depression for a love not returned. For those like me, who came from a college, it was easy to fall hopelessly in love with classmates. I stayed infatuated with the girl who smiled at me on the first day of school for the three years of high school, only with very short and superficial distractions. Nothing could be done to change that, but even today when I run into my old friends from high school, I reflect that the friendship from high school (with at least some classmates) remains for life. This friendship has the same complicity, the same spirit the same desire to laugh and make fun of the world. Although forty-five years later, many are parents or even grandparents, we still see the girl with cotton socks and a plaid skirt — or a boy with jeans and the scooter 48 who was so cool in those years.

I arrived at the end of high school exams practically without even realizing it. I don't remember much about my school exams, but my memory is razor sharp when I remember a trip I took with my three best high school friends to the Lido degli Estensi. We took Franco's old Taunus and left towards a beautiful holiday that screamed with happiness. Pure happiness which however closed the age of games. Now began the age when it had to be put to use — the "spirit of the game."

When I decided to choose medicine, I never had doubts that I would get to the very profound depths. The question was: in what time frame? To the depths of where? On graduation? During the specialty? At the first publication? Well, it was immediately clear to me that in medicine there is no point of arrival and that once you choose that career - you become a perpetual student.

For the power conferred on me by the Dean, the Magnifico

Rettore, and by proxy of the Italian State I declare you a Doctor of Medicine and Surgery

Here I am. Five and half years after I joined the medical school, I find myself a doctor like him. Like my father and as my grandfather and great grandfather. These are incredible moments. Emotion, satisfaction, and joy for my parents. Disbelief and mental confusion for my part in the face of this declaration by the Magnifico Rettore and my new existential condition.

I am a doctor and will be for a lifetime. There will be people who will entrust me to their problems and diseases. I will have to be the comfort and relief of so many individuals who believe in what I do and in what I represent. There we are. I will have to live up to the expectations and it will no longer be how to face an exam or written test, but rather, it will be real life. It will be all the more difficult and at the same time more important. The seasons of the game are over and there is no room for lightness or light heartedness. If I have a spare minute, I will have to devote this to science and improve my knowledge. This is what the Hippocratic oath asks. But I will also have to convince everyone that life is precious and that it must be lived with happiness and joy. Life is what I will have to preserve by accomplishing the mission that some call work, but that in the end, it is a challenge — a game, a game with disease and death. It is no longer the time for games, but the doctor must keep the spirit of the game to escape depression and contamination of depression when you are surrounded by the suffering and despair of your patients. Sometimes, and sometimes often, you see them die. The spirit of the game is that it must give you the strength to be cheerful even when there is no joy. It allows you to leave a room that has been touched by death and then proceed to meet with a couple with a smile after they have just welcomed a new life. A spirit that will make you seem serene talking to a seriously ill patient, even when you are deeply troubled and give you the strength to console him with real words. A game in which a life will pass away in your arms and a new discovery will save a hundred more lives. A game where the search for knowledge continues to push and inspire you to give hope for thousands of people. A game that you play by faith (profide) or by profession. And I will have to show myself as an optimist and positive as when we rejoiced as children for simple games of childhood.

As a doctor, I will be a playmate for the patient in the wonderful path of life where there are those who win and those that lose, but ultimately, we all come to the same end. The important point is to get there well, and possibly without pain. I will have to transmit trust and serenity even when Mother Nature will become unkind and dispense sufferings and diseases. Sometimes it will be difficult. Sometimes I may have to be a little adsorbed in my own thoughts to avoid giving painful answers. More often, I need to be ready with a joke to avoid my patients drowning in their own despair. It is necessary for me to remain connected as a little child and never forget the importance of the game, even if from now on it will be the game of life.

Lifestyle

My UNIVERSITY PATH ended with my degree and I had to give up my academic career for a series of reasons that mainly had to do with survival. A sick father, little money and the need to earn. I couldn't afford to have "crickets" on my mind. I absolutely needed to find a job to live, support my family and create my own pathway.

I was 25 when I left the University and left with regret. I promised myself to settle accounts with academia at another time in my life. After the state exam, I attended the hospital daily from Vicenza but worked without pay. One day an accountant that I had known for years from the "Ordine dei medici" (College of Physicians) asked if I wanted to replace a doctor for three days at a town near Vicenza. After a thousand uncertainties and self-doubts I declared myself available thinking that in such a short time, nothing serious could happen. I showed up in the clinic on a Thursday morning and found over 20 people waiting for me. All but two accepted to be visited by the young unknown doctor and I immediately embarked on a series of visits, injections and prescriptions.

In the three days and three nights that followed — everything that could happen — did, from acute appendicitis to home deliveries of new babies, serious pneumonia and pediatric diseases. Since I had seen most of these already from my hospital experience, I treated the patients (to the amazement of the villagers) without the necessity of a hospital recovery.

Less than a week had passed when a new proposal came for another 15-day substitution. The ice had clearly broken, and I felt almost like a veteran. I began traveling the hill towns in the area with my "Cinquecento" and honking as I approached, in much the same manner as my father with his "Topolino C" (a very small car) in the mountains. Those were hard days and sleepless nights. There were no medical backups (guardia medica) and my closest ally was the midwife, who in the case of home deliveries, acted in isolation.

I looked after children, parents and grandparents. I learned to listen to disputes between spouses and to solve problems of coexistence between neighbors. They asked me to help deal with difficult situations. I had to communicate to a father that his 18-year-old daughter was pregnant, but seven months later, that same father (now a grandfather) asked me to be the godfather of the child. It was also a difficult task to try and not institutionalize a mentally ill family member, but in the end the family was grateful to me to have spared him being imprisoned and isolated in a psychiatric institution.

I also have memories of Edoardo, the first child that I delivered, of Mr. Marco who needed to be hospitalized urgently for an acute appendicitis and the warm memories of moments shared with the people from the village. Some patients invited me to dinner as an important guest, others like I was part of the family. I have close ties with many and still today some send me thoughtful gifts, such as "Mary of the rabbits" that still sends me a gift basket brimming with good things to eats every Christmas. This is because for her, I am her doctor — period.

At the end of my experience, I found the teaching of my father had been confirmed. The village doctor has to deal not only with the "evils" of the body but also those of the soul. Success in life does not depend only on fate, but rather what you do and how you use your experiences. I went back to the hospital with an important experience that benefited myself

— but also others. Thanks to those days in the countryside, I believe that my patients today have a better doctor.

Exactly twenty-eight years after I was born, on even the same day in the middle of summer, my son Federico was born, and I became a dad. From this day forward a person counted on me, not only for a diagnosis or a cure, bur for everything: to eat, sleep warm, be safe, live a good life and possibly play. A newborn child cannot play and I — with a little impatience to start, began to look at him, to understand him in order to interact with him. I am happy that aunts, relatives and friends brought all sorts of games to Federico. While we were preparing the cradle in the bedroom of the house and hanging pendants and toys on the bars of the colored bed, my mind flashed back to when my grandmother told me about the cradle that they had prepared for me. Bicycle spokes and metal supports from an umbrella had been planted around it with wool balls, pompoms and remnants of socks. When the bar was touched, my gaze would be captured by the movement of the colored balls touching one another and making a cheerful ringing sound. Today there are literally thousands of toys for early childhood and I, in a few days of paternity have already become an expert on pacifiers, rattles and especially the bee carillon. This is a fantastic invention which consists of a steel bow that holds a swirl of paper mâché bees that move over the head of the bed to varied music. When I look at Federico I am captured by this and I look both at the bees that turn tirelessly and my son watching the bees. I could do this for hours. Becoming a father made me grow and feel even more adult and responsible, but it didn't deprive me of the taste for the game. Indeed, from today I have the pleasure of a new playmate in Federico.

The American Dream

On July 4, 1958 I was only 6 years old, but I still remember the emotion when I heard the notes of the American Anthem that filled the air for Independence Day. My father and I had been warmly welcomed in the American barracks of the Vicenza Military base ever since he had treated their injured during a military exercise at Asiago. I admired their attention facing the stars and stripes of the flag and the respect the soldiers had for all the commanders of the base. The joy of seeing these young proud Americans deeply affected me. I saw in them something I liked. I had a vague idea of America: stories from emigrants that had returned home or odd bits of news from the radio or pages from newspapers. In the middle of the square with the flags waving on the flagpole, I felt intimidated and curious. Would I ever go to America during my life? Difficult, I thought.

Ten years later in 1968, while Scott McKenzie was singing about San Francisco and how welcoming California was, swarms of young Italians took to the streets protesting about everything and especially against Americans. "Yankee go home" was their motto outlined in the marches of students against the war in Vietnam. Even on those occasions, I never managed to be part of the pack and indeed — the more that the "pack mentality" increased, the more I wanted to get out. I recognized that the US was not there making a good impression with the veterans returning home from Vietnam physically and psychologically destroyed. It wasn't the ideology that guided me, just good common sense and a desire to believe in a better world. When I enrolled in Medicine, I found myself in the middle of the anti-American protest movement stuck between anatomy exams and physiology interviews. The fact however was that any innovation, any interesting publication and all our books came from the United States. It was destiny. America with its contradictions continued to wink at me. One day Professor Andres from Buffalo, came to teach a lesson in the legendary Morgagni room of the University of Padova. I was struck by the modus comunicandi and the rhetorical "verve" of the professor that had literally become an immunopathology legend. I had an illumination. I understood that if one wanted to lead the way in our world that a stop in the USA was inevitable. Maybe for just a short time, but it had to be done.

***

Only after about thirty years and many internships/stages and various experiences, that eventually became solid paid work, I reached a certain tranquility and felt I could start looking around for something more permanent. I specialized in nephrology. Little Federico filled me with joy, but I still felt something was missing in my life and career. Early on, I realized the enormous competence of my colleagues in the Nephrology Department at the Vicenza hospital. They had vast and superior knowledge to those of university teachers. I convinced the group to write a book on the topic of dialysis which cost us a lot of work and sleepless nights, but which after about two years gave us recognition as excellent specialists in the field. It was time to make a quantum leap and we decided to organize an international conference on nephrology by inviting some of the world experts. In the meantime, I had cultivated a passion and study for hemofiltration, a technique that few knew well, and in a short time, I was considered a good expert.

I still felt however that I was missing something which

came when my boss found a scholarship for a willing doctor to do a three-month internship in America. There was no discussion in the ward. Everyone knew about my American dream, and moreover that experience in a world so different and far away was a little scary and at least some colleagues were also glad that it was I who led the way. I took a course in accelerated English conversation with a professor from British Vicenza School. I also prepared Federico who was still little, with a kind of calendar with windows because in the three-month absence, he could open a window each day and find indications for a treasure hunt that would lead to him earning either a chocolate or a toy. I didn't want him to feel abandoned. On Oct 25, a rainy day, I left Malpensa with Alitalia flight AZ600 to reach the heart of the United States — Manhattan. Juan, a colleague that had previously visited Vicenza to learn a new neonatal cure developed by me, was waiting for me.

The arrival in New York had been a little adventurous because in addition to the delays required by immigration for people that entered with a study visa, my American colleague had also left the car keys in the trunk of his car. To recover them, it was necessary to call a friend (that just happened to be a repentant car thief). In the Big Apple, everything seemed out of proportion and complicated. I had the determination however of a marine that lands on a beach infested with enemies. I could not dare waste those ninety days that could have been the first and even last of my American Experience. I had a precise budget and I knew how much I had to spend per day to keep a roadmap that would guarantee that I didn't end up sleeping under a bridge on the streets or starving.

My arrival at the hotel was dramatic. If you think of modern America as a sparkling large metropolis, you have the same idea that I had at that time, and the same disappointment I felt when I entered the Whales Hotel on Madison Avenue. Old and dirty with a crazy stale smell. I thought that it was for the cheap price you paid, but all things considered, it really wasn't very cheap: $150 day. The first night I slept in my clothes because the sheets were full of crumbs and hair. The floor was covered with a sage colored carpet and it creaked at every step for the presence of the cockroaches that shared the room. It was impossible to stay there. Luckily after a few days a patient of mine found me a small room at a pretty fair price

I worked day and night. I studied medicine, nephrology and English. In the hospital, they were kind enough which at least by New York Standards meant that I had to "make do." I had conquered a corner of the laboratory and I had delimited it with books and notebooks, so that the territory could be considered mine. My mentor, Juan was not only a doctor, but also extraordinary research scientist. He was Chilean in origin, but naturalized in the USA after marrying Peggy, a girl from New Jersey that couldn't be more American. All in all, he was a New Yorker and I was getting used to it. I was opening my mind to new and endless horizons. I collected everything and learned everything for fear of never again having this opportunity. One day Juan asked me to give a lecture, and since I had no slides or transparencies I spoke with gests and my broken English, helped by drawings with chalk on an old blackboard. I had studied physics and chemistry applied to dialysis and at that moment, I knew more about this than anyone that listened to me. They were amazed and concluded that the Italian "did have a head" and knew things they didn't know. They began to treat me like one of them. At the end of the three months they asked me to remain in America to work. My dream had been realized far beyond my initial expectations. Things were complicated however, and I decided to return to Vicenza.

My life in Vicenza was never the same as before. I had learned a new way to speak, to express myself and to think as the Americans. I dreamed in English and read the New York Times. Thus, began a period of prolific scientific articles which were published in national and international prestigious journals. The following year, Robert Bartlett, the father of Extracorporeal Membrane Oxygenation (ECMO) invited me to Ann Arbor Michigan to present the results of our clinical application of a device invented by me that allowed safe dialysis for children. We treated a girl from Puerto Rico, Esperanza, who had severe lung and kidney damage. Bob used my technique to support the kidneys, and his for the lungs. Together we saved that little girl. It was done. The following year I was invited to Cleveland, then the Mayo Clinic and the list of invites kept getting longer. Since I had been in America, they invited me at least 7-8 times a year and really treated me as an American that was occasionally lent to Italy. I had an even greater emotion when I was invited to give the keynote lecture at the 1992 American Society of Nephrology Congress.

In 1997, I was next in line to replace my boss in my historic department of Vicenza, when the law changed and allowed my boss to stay in charge for another 5 years. I was not very happy about being just an assistant, as I was forced to operate in conditions that were less than ideal. Sometimes I was the esteemed professor that was invited to international seminars, sometimes I was immersed and overwhelmed in the day-to-day activities of the hospital with three night shifts a week.

A solution finally arrived in 1998 when the American Medical Association award for the doctor and researcher that made the highest contributions to kidney patients over the decade of 1988-1998 was given to me. The award was named after Belding Scribner, the inventor of dialysis. It was given to me by the president of the association together with Nathan Levin, a colleague from New York who had created a research institute in Manhattan. On that occasion, Nathan asked me to come to America as a professor and director of his New York research laboratory. It was as if blue sky had suddenly exploded before my eyes. I talked at length with Paola, my wife, until I ran out of possible reasons for not accepting. In the end, we decided that we would be living in New York for the next two years. I had a huge amount of unused vacation days, so I could ask the Vicenza Hospital for a leave of absence. Although my boss wasn't overly enthusiastic, he also couldn't deny this opportunity as it was partially related to his prolonged work due to his missed retirement.

We only had six months to prepare for departure. Paola started the activities to leave our Italian home and make the necessary preparations for her parents, while I took care of Federico. Federico was 19 and was ready for us to spend a long period overseas. My enthusiasm couldn't be contained. I was finally going to live the American dream that I had since I was a student or apprentice and no longer as an occasional guest or supervisor, but as a full professor with an extraordinary assignment and a good salary!

***

We arrived in New York on a Friday evening and slept at the Hilton for a couple of days before entering our apartment on 95th Street. We went to IKEA and in two hours bought the furniture that would be with us for the next two years. My work colleagues were great. They had prepared an office overlooking downtown with two secretaries and a group of researchers that I would meet every Monday. The first week I was a little tense about doing a good job, however after 15 days I had everything in the palm of my hand. After four months we submitted a series of studies to the Congress of the American Society of Nephrology that pleased both the Dean and Hospital Administrator to the point, during a special dinner, that they gave me even more responsibilities and asked me to manage a chain of fifty-four dialysis centers distributed across the United States. In our New York Institute, companies were eager to collaborate with us, test their devices and collect our impressions.

Paola and I lived in an oasis of happiness. Federico often came for visits and we were so happy to be American in all respects. Without even realizing it, every time we traveled, at the end of short stays in Italy, we always said we were going back home. In New York we passed two beautiful Christmases, with the lighting of the tree, Macy's, and shopping.

For the last day of the millennium, we went to dinner at Windows on the World, the famous restaurant on the 125th floor of the south tower of the World Trade Center. To get there, we crossed Times Square where more than 2 million people were packed into the square since 4:00 p.m. waiting for the millennial passage. Fortunately, the dreaded Millennium bug never arrived, and everything went well. In fact, even my hospital buzzer never vibrated for emergency calls that evening.

We inaugurated the new millennium with a magnificent winter holiday in Florida, then a full immersion in the job: teaching at Albert Einstein College of Medicine. I couldn't be more satisfied. My course lectures were well attended, and it was a fruitful year for publications. September 16th I was invited for lunch at the 11 Madison restaurant by the Dean of the faculty, Nathan and Beth Israel Medical Center CEO. After a welcome drink and without further compliments, they asked me to stay at the University as a permanent faculty member and director of the research laboratory. The offer stunned me. It was extraordinary from both a professional and economic point of view. I asked for some time to talk to Paolo, Federico, and my boss from Vicenza. Within one week the general manager of the Vicenza hospital rushed to New York to meet me. He had understood everything. Lacking a counter-offer he would have difficulty asking me to give up on the Beth Israel Medical offer that would have been the crown on my American dream. He simply and clearly told me "Claudio, if you return you will be the new director of the Vicenza Nephrology Department. I will give your boss a strategic assignment. I'll organize the position opening before he even goes to retirement, which means that in a year from now, you will take his place. In the meantime, I will let you come to America when you want. In addition, we will start building a new futuristic department in Vicenza just as you want it." The offer could not have been more attractive. At the end of 2000, I returned to Italy and everything went as promised.

From that point I did return to America hundreds of times, always with much nostalgia. But I want to point out that my thoughts are not regret, but on the contrary, I can embrace the best of the two continents, America and Europe and take the best of what they can offer me. Of course, many mornings, looking at myself in the mirror before facing a full day of paperwork and mess, I wonder why I had not stayed in America, but I am so busy that I usually don't even have time to reply. My son did an internship in cardiology in Los Angeles. We have many friends in the United States and I am a member of several American scientific societies. Many consider me the most American of the Italians. Here in my country, I have tried to bring some America to Italy. Maybe I did it. Between a thousand difficulties and a thousand problems. But even today those who enter our department remark that it doesn't seem to be very "Italian." I take it as a great compliment and I realize that the American dream that I have cradled in my heart and mind could be realized even here in Italy where it was perhaps more difficult to achieve, but that is also what made it more incredible and wonderful.

Language and use

My father always said that those who know languages have the world in their hands. Unfortunately, there weren't many opportunities in Asiago to learn languages other than the dialect that we spoke at home and in the town square. Ours was a classic Venetian dialect, but with accents and inflections that varied from town to town and, in Asiago, even between neighborhoods. When I went down to Vicenza to attend the gymnasium, my companions made fun of me for my lilting accent that was typical of the "Altopiano." In no time though, I took on the cadence from Vicenza and you could hardly recognize where I had spent my childhood. Anyway, every time that I was over the last bend in the "Costo Road" to go back up to my mountains, my native accent of the Asiago square returned with unequivocally declared that I belonged to my small neighborhood within the community with the larger community of the area. During my University years I was able to easily acquire the Paduan cadence, which while at my first "condotta" (the family doctor job in a designated area) within the municipality of Cornedo that people thought I was originally from the Valle dell'Agno.

Regarding foreign languages — I can tell a completely different story. In the middle school of Asiago, we had a teacher who actually was quite poor in French. I remember nothing of her lessons, except for the one detail. She came to school with one NSU Prinz 1000. She drove it using normal low shoes, then quickly changed to elegant high heels before exiting the car. The consequence was that during the next two years of college I could barely make a mark of more than two out of ten. My mother, with good intentions sent me over and over to a teacher so beautiful that I could not stop looking at her, while my French did not improve at all. Moral: It seemed like my penchant for languages was poor and that I would have had anything but the world in the palm of my hands (as my father said). I still have difficulty with French today, not only for my bad initial start, but also because I have had few opportunities to practice it and have never shared much of a shared bond with the French people I know. I grimace at International congresses, where English is the official language and they do not renounce to speak in French. Some Gallic colleagues have confessed that the French government has subsidized participation at congresses on the condition that they present their work in French.

As for English, despite having a real passion for everything from America until I was about thirty years old, I sang songs from the Beatles by heart without understanding anything. When my American dream really began to materialize, and I received the communication regarding the scholarship in America, I threw myself in a frantic race to learn English. Mrs. Chatterton took pride in my progress and gave me compliments for the ultra-fast course that I completed in three weeks. Nevertheless, when I arrived in New York, the impact was devastating. I didn't understand a word. Day and night, I followed TV and radio to learn as much as possible. I first learned to express myself decently, then concentrated on understanding the local speakers. After a month, I went to Boston for a convention and a policewoman asked me if I was from New York. She said I had "caught their accent." So, I found out that in America it is not so different than Asiago. Cadences are important and tell where you are from. Upon returning from the USA, I also understood another thing. You really don't know a language by its lexicon, or some particular rule of grammar and syntax, but rather when you can express a concept in a manner similar to a native speaker.

Some people even made fun of me whenever I returned to Italy and couldn't think of the word or phrase in Italian. It was not a joke or an arrogant attitude. I simply had been so ingrained within the American world that I became estranged from my own origins. Over the years I have mastered English in such a way that I speak English in England with a certain cadence, in the US another (or more than one if I pass from New York to Los Angeles) and in Australia with an even different accent. For all countries use a language we call in jargon "Euro English" which is nothing more than an academic English that is well suited and can be understood by the Greeks, French, Polish and Spaniards. About the Spaniards, I confess that I have a love for their language as strong as my aversion for French. In the Iberian language, I do a total immersion at least one week per year when I walk along a section of the Camino de Santiago with friends and colleagues. I know Spanish enough to venture to speak it in their conferences, which has earned me their sympathy and facilitated my access to various Spanish and Latin American scientific societies. It actually seems to me that mine is a mixture of Spanish and Venetian dialect, but they say they can understand me and that I speak in perfect Castilian Spanish which obviously takes on an Argentinian cadence when I am in Buenos Aires.

Learning languages and speaking them is for me, a matter of respect for those who listen to you. Using the same language as the person that is speaking to you is a form of respect and demonstrates great civil spirit. This also applies, and is even more important, when communicating between a doctor and patient. It is reassuring for a sick person to hear a doctor speak with a clear and familiar language. I've always paid a lot of attention to the linguistic cadences of my patients to try and identify their origin and maybe also their social belonging so as to better connect with them and by adopting their accent to help them feel a bond or trust and make them feel at home. It is certainly important what we tell patients, but perhaps more important what they understand from our words. We must avoid too strong of a medical vocabulary filled with difficult terminology and complex details. It is enough to communicate the important information with simple, clear and transparent disclosure.

Giulietta, the passion of a lifetime

THE SUMMER OF 1958 was in full swing with a warm sunny holiday atmosphere. We had come down from the Altopiano by the Costo road and then went off through the Venetial countryside to Montebelluna, Treviso, the Terraglio road and finally to the lagoon and the entrance to the Lido. We were two families traveling in an old elongated "Millecento" with children on improvised small seats. At the bend of the river side, we stopped at a farmyard where they offered us fresh lemonade and some shade, while the driver was in a repair shop to vulcanize the tires. My father, generous as he was, always worried that we had enough to eat. He had discovered some fabulous skewered chickens at a nearby butcher and bought enough for an army. At half past noon, we sat under a grapevine pergola — shared with country farmers returning from the fields. We ate and drank with the taste of being together and the lightheartedness that only in those years I saw on people's faces. I was worried about our car and kept going around it as if my attentions could by magic bring the wheel back to its place and start it again.

I've always had a great passion for cars, fantastic objects that move on their own; ask you little and give you a lot. As a child, I was enchanted by the roaring monsters that darted during the Mille Miglia at night and, like all children, I collected model cars. I had a whole box. The two jewels in my collection were a Lancia Aurelia B24 and an Alfa Romeo Giulietta Spider. My favorite was of course the Giulietta Spider.

Finally, the driver returned with the wheel properly

repaired and balanced and our adventurous journey resumed. The scent of the sea salt hit us as soon as we crossed the bridge over the silo. It seemed to me that I could already see our coveted beach. Our joy as children was irrepressible when we arrived at the small "Pensione Amelia" which seemed even more modest near the majestic Hotel Bagni and Miramare.

In those years, Jesolo was a mirror of post-war Italy, animated by a great desire to live and progress. Craftsmen and industrialists were beginning to have enough profits to send their wives to the best hotels by the sea. Evenings were spent dancing and clubs began to be frequented by clientele who could actually afford a few bottles of champagne. New cars circulated on the roads. There was the Topolino and the Seicento, but also cars that were more than a million lire — or even three million lire, like Ferraris and Porsches. Usually these appeared in Jesolo on Sunday when the new rich came to find their wives on vacation. I had a favorite bench in via Bafile, the street parallel to the promenade, where I sat for hours, swinging my legs that didn't even touch the ground, watching the cars that paraded in front of me on display. I described and cataloged all the models in a notebook. I had also drawn up a ranking of common, rare and unique models. Among the rare ones was the American Thunderbird, among the German models was the Opel Kapitan that stood out for its almost American design. Small, three-wheeled cars and large Mercedes cars passed in front of me, popular cars like the Trabants that came from the East and elegant cars like the Lamborghini or Maserati, but above all was the new Alfa Spider, the Giulietta. It was my love and every time it passed on the avenue, I envied the drivers, middle aged gentlemen or privileged children accompanied by female beauties worthy of the wonderful car. The colors were the canonical ones of the Giulietta — a white, halfway between white and cream; a sky blue reserved for only a few specimens because it was initially designed for the Bertone coupe, the Giulietta Sprint, and of course — red. Not any red, but a "non-red" that was slightly orange red which changed according to the hours of the day and the reflections of the sun. Almost orange in the morning, at sunset it took on tones of a deep burgundy red. This color had been wanted by Sergio Pininfarina himself who had not like the "classic" Alfa red for "his" Giulietta Spider. When I thought of a Giulietta without having it in front of my eyes, the image that materialized in my mind was always colored in Pininfarina red.

I would sit for hours on the bench, swinging my legs and waiting for a leap in my heart when the unmistakable silhouette of the Giulietta spider would loom on the horizon. I appreciated the nose that looked out from afar with the two headlights like intelligent and curious eyes, the Alfa Romeo shield as cheeky as a French nose, and underneath, the two "moustaches" of the plates that made me think of a kind of open mouth with a perennial smile. I liked its streamlined and slender profile with the wraparound windscreen and the soft top completely hidden in the compartment behind the seats. I like the little "round behind" with the two lights on the side tails that looked like the bright earrings of a mannequin. The license plate rose vertically from the chromed bumper like a warning sign saying" Hey, I'm Giulietta — don't dream of even touching me!." When I happened to find a parked Giulietta, I always stopped to check the steering wheel, the analog instruments — the tachometer and speedometer, the gear lever the vinyl leather seats (called skai), the Pininfarina frieze on the passenger's glove compartment. I mentally made a note of any different detail and immediately went to find out if it was an authorized or spurious variant. If it was the effect of an original personalization of the owner or the result of careless maintenance. One day, while I was biting a licorice popsicle on my bench, I saw six Giuliettas pass in less than an hour. Three red, one blue and two white. It seemed almost an insult to my passion, and at that moment I decided that when I grew up that I would have "my" Giulietta. One of the few surviving examples of a discontinued Giulietta model would become my jewel.

Over the years, Alfa Romeo continued to produce more or less important variants of the Spider until they finally turned the page and produced the Duetto. This also had several variations. One of them became famous because of the film *The Graduate* starring Dustin Hoffman. Having said that however, I remain surprised that some people exchange the Duetto for the original and unique Giulietta Spider. They have no idea what they are talking about! It would be like exchanging scorzone for the Alba truffle or a cheap ham for the prized culatello or a cheesy parmesan for one from the mountains or a pathetic margarine for a malga butter — produced in the best months of the mountain pasture. They are as different from each other as China is from America. In the meantime, I had graduated and started my internship with a salary of one hundred and twenty five million lire a month. The Giulietta remained in my dreams, but I certainly could not have crickets in my head, also because I was newly married and my wife earned less than me. We also were expecting our first child, Federico, occupying all our thoughts and concentration. But I continued to track every time an article, photo or comment appeared in print and put these together in a special notebook, together with scientific articles, energy bills and mortgage notes. In the second half of the nineties, I went more often to the United States where I was quite appreciated and well compensated for my work, my research and teaching activities in the field of nephrology. My good friend, Gianfranco from Vercelli, owned an old Mercedes 190 and a Jaguar E-type and continued to tempt me with offers of vintage cars including a Triumph, an MG and a Jaguar. But apart from the fact that the British — as I called them - were machines not suitable for my wallet, I also considered them as "terrible ferrivecchi" or old "rust bucket." They were unreliable and easy to leave you standing as they died at the first corner turn. When I emigrated to the USA to hold a professorship at the Albert Einstein University in the Bronx, I had a fabulous salary and royal treatment - just to continue with the research that I had previously carried out in secret during the downtime of my hospital duties.

Paola and I had found a home in New York. On a Saturday in March of the year 2000, I remember it exactly, as we went to Soho by bicycle to have lunch with our friend Paolo on Spring street. We were sitting at the corner table between Spring and Thompson when I received a call from Gianfranco: "Claudio — he tells me — I found your Giulietta. To tell the truth, it is not in great shape, but there are many pieces and it won't be difficult to rebuild and bring it back to life." Since the price was not too bad, I decided with both feet on the ground to buy the ailing car. I would have him put it into a warehouse waiting to start the restoration once we returned to Italy and realizing it would take time. Months passed and I only had photos of "my" Giulietta — dismembered elements, the two bumpers, a dashboard, a hood, wheels and a box with various pieces that once assembled, would have made up the engine.

In the summer, the Director General of the Vicenza hospital had come to visit me in New York and had promised me a soft return with a guaranteed position as the department chief. I returned to Italy in December. What an alienating impression to pass on a night of harsh winter from the blazing New York illuminations to the faint and almost invisible light of the streetlamps from my city! The days of return were intense and excited. There was a lot to do after two years absence. Paola's work, home and parents to be accommodated; friend and colleagues to re-establish contacts. Federico and his school. Lots to do. But after fixing everything my thoughts continually went to the old garage with the rusty shutter that contained the relic of my Giulietta. The time had come for the restoration of my red fireball — or rather Pininfarina orange red to begin.

The first phase, boring but necessary, was a general census of the present and missing pieces. In the following months, with the list in hand, we began to scavenge exhibitions and fairs of vintage cars and to plunder warehouses and auto parts in search of the original steering wheel, the two-tone trumpets produced by the historic FIAMM, the emblem with the primitive writing "Alfa Romeo Milan" which would later become only "Alfa Romeo," up to the original screws of the wiper blades. For a well-done restoration, you have to turn to professionals. I was lucky enough to find the Tecchio family, Catterino and Andrea, father and son, who knew about the Alfa Romeo. They had a workshop on the road in Bertesina. Cars accumulated in their courtyard, waiting repair or occasionally, valuable vintage cars would arrive. Almost always there was an Alfa Romeo of the carabinieri destroyed or some old model of the house of Arese without the engine or with the bodywork gutted. Inside the workshop there was a collection of memorabilia, models, photos and memories of cars that had raced the Mille Miglia or had an important past. Engine parts and body parts were scattered everywhere. One day Catterino said to me in a cheerful manner "Dr Ronco, I bought a scrap car to rebuild your Giulietta, but before we start the work (which will be long), you must tell me one thing. Are we restoring a Giulietta to sell to the first buyer hoping to get a good deal, or reviving a car to be jealously preserved for years to come? You know in both cases the method, work and expenses are completely different"

"Catterino," I answer him "I have been waiting for this moment for years. This will be "my" Giulietta and I will never separate from it again. We will never part."

"So go on" Catterino exuberantly told his son. They were happy to have found a person who shared their passions. The first job fell to the body worker, Anselmo. The car had to be stripped bare. I went to see the progress twice a week. With a circular cutter, Anselmo worked on the oxidation points until he met a layer of clean metal without rust. Sometimes the sheet was so thin that he risked piercing it, but it was only in this way that one could be sure that the rust would not resurface in the future under the paint, just to deform and dent the metal again. After several weeks the perfectly polished body was re-assembled, and the holes were covered with an anti-rust filler. In the case of "more serious" injuries, as analogous in the hospital for a human body torn by trauma, Anselmo had welded patches of a new metal sheet by filling and then milling until a perfectly smooth surface was obtained. This went on for months. Catterino had told me "let's not go on rebuilding the mechanical parts and the engine until we are sure we can have good bodywork."

In the meantime, we started the process for the paperwork for the new plates. The department of motor vehicles warned me that it was not going to be an easy task. In fact, the procedure for unlocking the car registration and plate numbers, and therefor of the car itself needed to go to a type of publication in the public automobile registry with an accompanying new registration application. Although some things seemed simple enough (returning the old registration and plates), the registration couldn't be made until after the car was tested, and the testing was only possible after the vehicle was completed. It would certainly be some time before I would see the light at the end of the tunnel.

The bodywork proceeded by hard dedicated manual work that included leveling the surface with sandpaper. Sometimes stucco had to be added to the patch points to fill in the small differences in height with the rest of the bodywork. It was then necessary to wait for the new layer to consolidate before continuing with the sanding, always by hand since the electric sander could detach the new patches. Before the actual color, several coats of primer were applied in very thin layers to make sure they adhered perfectly. Once everything was dry, they finished the surface with 400 grit water sandpaper.

The painting day was particularly exciting. It was a unique satisfaction to see that orange-red color that we had requested from the Pininfarina warehouses and that had been sent to us in half kilo jars, as if they were vials of vin santo. To see the paint that came out of the spray gun was nothing less than extraordinary. I let Anselmo complete his work and at six in the evening, I went back to the hospital to follow a patient who had presented some problems. This was also because "my" Giullietta would need to stay in the paint oven for a few days.

Finally, the big day arrived. The complete body and all its parts arrived on a truck at Catterino's shop, ready to be unloaded. The Giulietta was lowered with a small crane and placed on four wooden supports. Catterino and Andrea put their hands in their hair and exclaimed "oh my God! What did Anselmo do?! With all of his experience, how could have painted the engine compartment and the trunk of a 1958 model in anti-noise black?" There was a moment of absolute panic and I realized that the car would not be reborn in the following weeks, but that it would take other months to restore the internal compartments to that red paintwork that was required by the sacred register of the historical Alfa Car reports as the only and authentic way that a 1958 Giulietta model could be. It was therefore, reloaded on the same truck and disappeared in the fog of the Vicenza winter. A couple of months later, the ceremony was repeated and this time we were happy to uncork a bottle of prosecco to celebrate the beginning of the mechanical work on a perfect body. It was also the beginning of a series of long discussions and friendly encounters (and clashes) with Catterino and his son for technical inconveniences that delayed the work and for some distraction of my trusted mechanics during the long moths of the restoration.

For a year and a half, we worked on the preparation of the frame with the axels, the steering unit, the differentials and the springs with leather straps as the original model. Everything had to be original, down to the very last particular detail. The work on the engine was particularly interesting. The structure was originally made of steel and it could have degraded over time, Catterino wisely suggested a nitriding process in which each part of the engine was subjected to a galvanic bath which made the metal surface practically indestructible. Each day was a marvel to see the progress as I passed by the Tecchio shop after my work in the hospital. Every piece of scrap metal that came out of the box became beautiful and found its place on the engine block, which gradually started to take shape. Cylinders, connecting rods, valves, cylinder heads gaskets, oil pan, the distributor. At the beginning of the third working Spring, the engine was finally ready to be lowered into the hood compartment. Everything miraculously fell into place. It was now a matter of connecting the pieces with the rest of the equipment. The connection to the electrical system — incredibly simple, especially when compared to the control units of today's cars, was a trivial matter. The assembly of the instruments was a little more laborious and then we just couldn't get the tachometer to work. Finally, we were able to get a new tachometer in Modena at an antique market, while the original black and white steering wheel couldn't be found. To solve this, Catterino had the brilliant idea to take out of his archive the photo of a Giulietta from '58 equipped with a three-pronged wooden steering wheel. We found the same steering wheel in question at a market from Padua and assembled it without delay. It was now time to bring the car back to the body shop to mount the doors with the windows, the last seals and to check the support structure of the retractable hood on which the newly made-to-measure canvas was mounted. In the meantime, the seats had been completely renewed with imitation leather of the original colors. The only unorthodox detail, an electric pump for petrol was mounted so as not to drain the poor battery in an attempt to fill the carburetor when the car was stationary for several days. Finally, the big day for testing arrived. I was busy in the hospital and could not be present. Andrea had to take the car to the motor vehicle department in the morning where they would carry out the registration checks. I could hardly stand the wait of wanting to know how it went! I finally managed to leave the hospital and to the Tecchio shop only at eight in the evening. Catterino came up to me with his usual gruff voice and said frowning: "They gave you three plates, doctor." But what does that mean? Did I pass or not? Do I have the registration? Catterino with pride exclaimed "Your Giulietta has passed the exam with flying colors and has two shiny new plates together with the booklet to circulate. The third plate is the gold plate of the ASI (historic Italian Autoclub) that you can apply to the rear bumper as a guarantee of professional restoration." There was nothing more I could say, because everything, including a moment of shared emotion shared by Andrea, was overcome by the pop of a bottle of prosecco and the overflowing cheerfulness of Lidia (Catterino's wife) who sliced fresh salami for our improvised celebration.

It was the first of May, 2000 (Labor Day in Europe) for the baptism of "my" Giulietta. We were ready. I was driving with Paola by my side in our red "fireball." My wife jokingly asked, "Do I need to be jealous of this new young girlfriend of yours." I replied that I wouldn't really consider her so young considering that she was still almost fifty years old. I started taking the direction of the Riviera of the Brenta up to that famous bridge over the silo beyond which I saw my previous visual landmark of my first trip as a boy: Jesolo. Running up and down via Bafile, I enjoyed the stroll with my two friends and deep loves — Paola and Giulietta. Suddenly, right near the famous access to the sea, near the Hotel Bagni and Miramare, I saw the bench of my youth and I noticed a 5 or 6 year old boy sitting there with his legs dangling and a notebook in his hand watching cars go by. "Could it be…? Naaah!"

III. Time for Responsibility

"Twenty years from now you will be more disappointed by the things that you didn't do than by the ones you did do."

—*Mark Twain*

The Connectivist

IT ISN'T EASY to collaborate with people, nor make people collaborate, especially in a job where there are different personalities, competencies, and habits. Each person is committed to asserting his own vision and solutions. Ever since childhood however, I always tried to foster a spirit of collaboration — especially when games between friends would often degenerate into sometimes violent clashes. At the University, it was easy for me, as a half-revolutionary and half-model student to make assertions that could be accepted by professors. I consider the positive compromise when the synthesis of different modalities can result in a common interest. On the other hand, I detest it when it is the fruit of ignorance and subterfuge.

I have always had a strong interest in a particular organ of the human body — the connective tissue. Its function is to essentially hold together organs and tissue of different types in a kind of compartmentalized box, where each can find its place and perform its function. Connective tissue was not always recognized as its own "real" organ with supporting characteristics, homeostatic cushioning, hormonal functions and immune defense. My interest in this theme dates back to 1964 when, reading the science fiction classics of the time, I came across a book by Alfred E. van Vogt entitled: *The Voyage of the Space Beagle*. The book was about a spaceship engaged in an interstellar mission. There were several scientists on board who had to conduct a series of experiments. The crew included a chemist, an engineer, a doctor and a botanist.

There were also sociologists, psychologists, veterinarians, and computer scientists. The cream of science of a somewhat advanced terrestrial civilization. There was however a particular scientist, Dr. Grosvenor, who had no specific skills. His function was to bring together the knowledge of different scientists and to give a sense of "unity" or completeness to the series of experiments that otherwise could not have given rise to useful applications for humanity.

Entering later in the world of medicine and science, I realized that the different disciplines each proceed on their own in parallel tracks without necessarily having a cross pollination or exchange of information or knowledge and that this was due in part to petty envy, but also to more substantial reasons such as the desire to control research funds or department funding. This resulted in a huge waste of resources and possibilities. The lack of osmosis between disciplines often leads to repeat experiments already carried out by others. In scientific research inclusion gives back more than exclusivity.

Even in medicine, as physicians, we often tend to place emphasis and attention on organs rather than the whole organism or "being" at the center of our attention and knowledge. It is like seeing a tree and not being aware of the forest.

Furthermore, or for lack of humility or common language, we, as physicians, tend to neglect to explore different disciplines from which we could draw many useful elements to our own work. For these reasons, for the early years of my career as a doctor and researcher, I set out to become a *"connectivist"* in the manner of Grosvenor.

In 1980, the nephrology department and the intensive care unit of the Vicenza hospital couldn't have been farther apart from each other — physically and conceptually. The two departments were housed in different buildings and each discipline had little or no contact in the treatment and approach towards the patients. In the five-year period from

1975 to 1980, we had fifty-five cases of acute renal failure, of which 90% had been diagnosed and followed by the nephrology department and 10% were managed by the ICU with a mortality of nearly 100%. In contrast, in the year 2000, there were 525 cases of which 87% had been managed by the ICU with a mortality of about 60%. What had changed in the twenty years to the different approach and outcome to acute kidney injury? Surely, it was greatly due to the collaboration between nephrologists and ICU doctors for the most critical patients. On my return from Mount Sinai Hospital in New York, I was able to convince them by pointing out that as the average age of the population rose, the critical patients would increase. In short, every doctor knows how to play their own instrument — but with a single instrument you can only play a simple melody. If you want to play a symphony, the instruments must be tuned to the same note. Thanks to a series of publications and training events organized by us on this treatment model, Critical Care Nephrology has been considered for some time as a real discipline and referred to as the "Vicenza Model." Today, any project launched at our Institute sees doctors, engineers, biologists, physicists, and pharmacists gathered at the same table. In addition, we include a health economist that is also employed and provides us with a real-time assessment of the cost/benefit ratio and sustainability of the project.

The doctors from our Nephrology staff visit the ICU, even when we are not called, and we now regularly find ourselves with our ICU colleagues even just for a coffee. We talk about our children, our common problems — from the mortgage to the need for a new car over a cappuccino and brioche. This has helped us get to know each other better and have an increase in mutual trust. Now in many cases, we do more prevention than cure and solve many problems before they arise or degenerate into more complex clinical scenarios. We created bridges between our specialties focusing on what we now call the "chat" or crosstalk between different organs.

With this in mind, we have created new classifications on cardio-renal, hepato-renal syndromes and on the interactions between the lung and kidney or the brain and kidney. How many things can be learned from different specialists! It is fantastic and above all, so nice to speak a common language also to the clinical engineer or pharmacologist.

Recently for example, we have focused on the use of biomarkers. These are molecules that the body produces under conditions of stress or developing damage. They are like red flags that appear in a patient's medical history and that can alert the attending physicians. With the Mayo team, we developed a several alarm systems called "electronic noses." These are algorithms or artificial intelligence systems capable of alerting the doctor in the presence of particular situations and with a very high predictive capacity. To be able to really benefit from biomarkers, you need to have computerized medical records that can connect the immense data today offered by international registries. It is incredible to think that the worldwide data generated from antiquity to the end of last year is the same amount of data generated in our international registry in two months! This is today what is known as "Datafication" or "big data." We are not speaking of megabytes, but rather of gigabytes (1000 megabytes), tetrabytes (1000 gigabytes), petabytes (1000 terabytes), exabytes (1000 petabytes), zettabytes (1000 exabytes).

How can we use so much data for real clinical utility? We often have more information than time to analyze it. We run the risk that doctors only look at the computer and not the patient. Again, it takes a "connectivist," but this time electronic. Artificial Intelligence, fortunately does not have cultural or ideologic barriers but will be the best way to avoid the dangers inherent in the lack of conscience of the machine. On the one hand, massive computerization can lead to an optimization of processes with the advantage of raising the standard of care for all patients, but it can also cause a type of massification of information and depersonalization of assistance. We should bear in mind that the standard is not the maximum goal to be achieved, but the lowest common denominator from which to improve. An individual is always at the center of action and interest of the doctor. For years now in Italy, and especially in Vicenza, we have been offering the privileged doctor-patient relationship and have insisted on personalizing treatments. Now the Americans have invented "precision medicine," a medicine based on the individual response to treatments, even planned based on the human genome, the only and final distinction between two individuals. We are experiencing a moment of great transformation in theories and practices of care. In our institute, we have created the school of Humanistic Medicine, so that nothing of the ethical relationship with the patient is lost. We want to teach our young doctors the importance of the individual patient and their history. We must prevent a machine from ordering the cure that knows nothing of the history of the patient, but we also can't neglect the enormous benefits and help that the machine can give us. It is up to us to receive and transform these suggestions into conscious actions and not to accept orders in subtle ways using the computer as a sterile surrogate for our brain. *Cogito ergo sum.*

Fortunately, I have been ill only a few times during my life and for the most part, I have waited for the illness to pass, trusting more in nature than medicine. However, when my problem was well defined and required medical attention, I lost my clear headedness and asked my doctors the same absurd questions that my patients continually ask me. The truth is when we are sick, we are fragile. We feel weak and helpless because we become prisoners of the disease that takes away our independence and quality of life. We, as doctors, are the least ready to be treated, since we are usually in the position to only treat and be in control. In my family, if there is no critical need such as the need for a heart transplant, I too will let everything resolve itself, while in the hospital for minor reasons I rush to make sure that the patient has all the assistance and care available. The patient is a person who loses points of reference and the ability to reason, and therefore, needs a tutor. That guardian is his doctor, who will also be his lawyer and confessor. I say this not to encourage a paternalistic view of care, but to make people understand the substantial difference between to cure and to take care. To cure someone, in a sterile manner is to face the illness regardless of who has the symptoms or suffers from it. Instead, to take care, is a way of making one's knowledge and objectivity available to the patient by exercising compassion.

How many times does the patient see the doctor as a detached judge who does not participate in his misfortunes and asks the doctor to put himself in his own shoes. Of course, if I had shared all the sufferings of my patients, I would have been dead for some time, but this doesn't mean that sometimes I can't or shouldn't become part of their emotion or get into their situation. Often, during morning rounds in the ward or in the clinical discussion meetings, I ask my collaborators who are sometimes uncertain of their decisions: "what would you do if the patient was your brother or sister or parent. Here, going beyond the signs and symptoms of the disease and trying to understand the needs of the subject. Their emotions and fears. To comfort their suffering is part of the cultural background of what we could now call the doctor 4.0. The new doctor must be able to juggle different modes of diagnosis: from purely observational to clinical with manual semeiotics, from nosographic diagnosis linked to clinical biochemistry to instrumental diagnosis based on new imaging techniques and up to incorporation of genetic and molecular information. But it also must be anchored to the humanistic dimension of the profession. You must live the mission. The new doctor is the one who is able to put himself in someone else's shoes at the moment of illness and need. This is the type of doctor that we would all like to have at our bedside.

Ethics and the art of being cured

IN MY LIFE I have always declared my intention to tackle the issues of medicine within a humanistic vision. That is, not only mathematics, physics, biology, anatomy. These all serve to make a good doctor, but also art, philosophy, poetry, history. The human sciences, which I prefer to call humanities to remove the perverse thought that inhuman sciences exist, are indispensable no less than the exact sciences for the optimal exercise of the medical profession. The doctor must study the patient and his condition first of all with the tools of anthropology, psychology and sociology. Only later, after collecting the history of the patient, can you move to a clinical hypothesis, a diagnosis and perhaps a prognosis. In all this ethics should not be forgotten. without an ethical approach, the dignity of the sick person cannot be safeguarded. Umberto Veronesi, on the occasion of a visit to our Institute, told us: "you cannot imagine an evolved humanism without moral values, and you cannot imagine a medicine without ethical values." Ethics is a vision of life that continually rediscovers the infinite possibilities of redeeming us, day by day, from any state of misery. Humanism also means much more: curiosity, wonder, amazement, research, design, trust in intelligence, art of knowing how to live and be in the world. Humanism teaches us to live the present well by capitalizing on the experiences of the past to design the future with passion and reason. Humanism and ethics, therefore, in function of the pursuit of the common good.

Ethics are not absolute, but this does not mean that we must fall into that relativism, abhorred by Benedict XVI, where everything can be called into question. Ethics should be a continuous question to act in a logic of progressive improvement. And the doctor's ethos, that is, his behavior, should be moral and shared. Each of us has a personal ethic, but none of us is an island, especially the doctor who has more social responsibilities than anyone else. Bearing the weight of responsibility means "knowing how to respond," being responsible for one's actions and one's way of being. This implies understanding, respect and indulgence towards those who have ideas and behaviors that contrast with ours. However, the ability to tolerate must not go beyond do-goodism and paternalism. The compassionate doctor kills the sick, recites an old proverb.

As a doctor I can say that the first tolerance must be towards ourselves, if only to avoid posing as (useless) heroes. We can't carry all the burdens of the world. It is enough to blame a few. The doctor must be able to accept the consequences of his decisions, aware that he takes these in stride to maintain a balance between courageous and defensive choices. Ethics, in fact, cannot be considered a normative science, since moral judgment is not based on objectively measurable elements, but on the sensitivity (and creative unpredictability) of people. It being understood that the conceptions of good and evil, good and right have changed and change according to the times and cultures. It is no coincidence that today, in the hospital, cultural mediation is often required for patients from countries other than ours that help the doctor not only understand their language but also and above, all their concepts, their customs, their traditions.

As Umberto Veronesi said, there are different types of ethics. There are lay ethics based on epistemology and religious ethics based on faith, the ethics of finance and the ethics of industry, the ethics of human relationships and medical ethics. But ethics in everyday medicine is an elusive concept. The first ethical foundation that should inspire a doctor's behavior is respect. Respect for the person, health, life, nature. The doctor should be a healer of the evils of the body and the evils of the soul because soul and body coexist in the greatest good that is life. The doctor is the priest of life and owes his patients every effort to make their life better. The good doctor is empathetic, cures, soothes, supports, supports, consoles. In a word he loves. To prevent the bureaucratic-administrative tasks that are increasingly numerous and heavy imposed on doctors by the modern model of care to the detriment of the care activities, result in a dehumanizing system, it is essential to place the patient at the center of care, make him a protagonist of the Department. In other words, the patient must feel part of a collective effort that has as its final result not only the solution of his disease problems but also an improvement in his level of health and quality of life. if the objective is the well-being of the patient, the care must be expertly modulated between the standards indicated in the international guidelines based on scientific evidence, and the specific needs of the patient. These high levels of attention of the caring staff have beneficial effects on the patient because they reinforce hope and yearning for a positive solution. Unfortunately, a happy ending is not always possible because it is not true, as modern media induce us to think, that everything is curable. There are chronic diseases, and there are also events such as the end of life, that sometimes occurs prematurely. But even in the presence of incurable disease or severe impairments, the ethical care model based on a strong "passion" leads the patient to feel that his pain is shared and divided among the members of a team (doctor and patient against disease and suffering: result of the ideal soccer game, two to zero), and if he does not earn in quantity of life, he earns in quality of life: one can spend the "rest of life" with less pain and more joys, even small, that deserve to be lived.

***

If the body is cared for by the "good" (ethics), the soul is cared for by the "beautiful" (aesthetics) with the advantage also of the body. There is no day, in my medical practice and in the exercise of my functions as director of a public service, that you do not meet me and "square-up" to the aesthetic dimension. For example, the occasion of an interview with a very kind and calm lady who is about to face a very serious problem. I must tell you that the husband with whom you have shared the last fifty-five years of your life is suffering from severe kidney disease and that you will soon have to undergo dialysis. I know the news will be devastating for these two people. While, amid a thousand doubts and hesitations, I am looking for the most delicate way to communicate it, I express my discomfort by mechanically stroking the smooth surface of the wall to which I am leaning with my hand. It is a damaged spot that I had repaired and repainted a few days ago. A wounded wall, like my patient who trusts me. How many things a peeling wall tells you! It can be the result of the lack of precision with which the bricklayer superimposed the bricks leaving overhangs and small imperfections that later became large cracks; or the haste that did not allow the mortar to dry at the right point; or a sloppy and superficial painting that has not eliminated bubbles and irregularities of the background with consequent detachments of paint. But even a perfect wall can have its ailments when every day they throw trolleys, furniture or various tools on it. Now if the progressive wear of a wall is physiological and understandable in a public environment where you run and grind hours and hours of activity, it is not acceptable that whoever passes in front of you does not see it or behaves as though he didn't see it. Of course, this wouldn't happen at home. The maintenance of a place is the mirror of those who live in it, and a well-kept or neglected wall in a hospital corridor also tells us how it can be the maintenance of an operating room, an ultrasound or a defibrillator. It is something that does not escape a patient and that in him translates into a greater or lesser trust in the medical and health personnel who have him in care and in a different level of anxiety or tranquility.

Today there are plenty of certified processes that help not only to remember when to repair, but also to document if and how the repair was performed. however, there is no certification that takes if carelessness and negligence become a rule or, worse, a lifestyle, as carelessness and negligence often demonstrate to places and monuments that make Italy's beauty. What is the cause? Certainly an excess of obtuse individualism that leads us to think that what is not ours is nobody's stuff. Or perhaps, overwhelmed by a thousand problems, we no longer feel the pride of beauty and the need for beauty. if we consider beauty not as an expression of chance or futile aestheticism, but as the result of attention, care and organization, we will find that beauty coincides with the good and the useful. Thus I think stroking the healed wall waiting to find the right words to tell my kind interlocutor that talking about the problem of your husband and the artificial kidney is more difficult than facing that problem in reality. "There will be difficulties - I say to the lady - but they will be overcome by facing them one by one. Once we died of this disease, today a dialysis can live a decent life, next to loved ones. Your husband and she will be welcomed by us as in a family and you will be followed in all phases of the treatment. We will start with a good planning and we will continue with a personalized prescription of the therapies and with a constant verification of the treatment in order to avoid complications ." In short, if your husband was a wall - I would like to tell you - and the care was the paint that covers it, we would do everything to ensure that the restoration is beautiful and good, and that subsequent maintenance will be of the same quality. In our department there will be no peeling walls or neglected diseases, there will be no crumbling or sick structures left to themselves. Carelessness and neglect are worse than ignorance or error, because they are the result of ignorance and mental misery and not the lack of resources, and people. In illness there is nothing beautiful, but a little beauty can help to cure or at least to live your sick state with greater serenity and hope.

Children are the best example of spontaneity and practicality. They tell you what they think and don't think about what they say. Children don't like ugly people and if you present them with a cute babysitter, they immediately love it. After all, when we are sick, we all go back to being children; we are afraid of evil, we say what we think without frills, and we want to suffer as little as possible. We don't like bad things either, while beautiful things make us feel better. And why not apply these concepts to those who are a little more children than we are, not by choice, but because suffering and disease made them such, fragile and in need of affection and beautiful things? Among the sufferings of a patient who arrives at the hospital, in addition to those directly related to his illness, which would be sufficient, there is a state of suffering induced by the estrangement of the environment, by the poor empathy of the people around him and by the perception to live a negative moment within what the Anglo-Saxons would call an unfriendly milieu: a hostile environment. In the collective imagination the environment of a private clinic is by definition clean and comfortable, the staff is qualified and with good presence, the nurses are nice; on the contrary, if the environment of the public hospital is perceived as sloppy, doctors, nurses and auxiliary staff scruffy in dressing and listless in acting. they are commonplaces that do not grasp the truth. The quality of an environment does not depend on whether it is public or private, which provides free or paid medical services, but on the human quality of those who work there and those who organize the service, starting from the boss. It is true that talking about leaders today in hospital seems like a blasphemy, given that the hierarchy of functions and responsibilities has been practically abolished by law and the professional figures are less and less differentiated. But in the end, you want for the authoritativeness of the indications of the Manager or you want for a spirit of emulation of the goodwill operators towards an apical figure of reference, the difference always makes the handle. So we remind the handle that if it wants to avoid a listless and cold service and an environment hostile to the sick, it must make organizational efforts that have a lot to do with aesthetics: the aesthetics of the care model, the aesthetics of the environments and the aesthetics of communication. My sociologist friend, Filiberto, author of many books on the subject, calls it "the aesthetics of the tertiary sector." The aesthetics of the rooms. It includes everything around the suffering individual. Flowers, paintings, elegant and practical architectural solutions, skillful alternations of colors, are elements that cushion the perception of pain and evil. "I don't even feel like I'm in the hospital," says someone staying in the colorful, airy and clean rooms of our ward. The aesthetics of the environment, contrary to what many think, does not require large investments. The maintenance of appliances, doors and trolleys that squeak to avoid annoying noise pollution are simple and inexpensive. Covering the walls with bright colors that are easy on the eye and cheer up the souls, as was done in the Vicenza Hospital in collaboration with the Polytechnic of Milan, costs nothing more than painting rooms and corridors with something other than the usual melancholy dirty white. To improve the aesthetics of our department, we have also created a small internal museum where objects, health devices, devices and innovations made by us in the last thirty years are exhibited. They have a historical-didactic function for the new generations of doctors and health workers, as well as entertainment for people forced to wait long times in those environments.

Even more important is the aesthetics of communication. How many and how different are the ways of communicating or explaining a situation by a doctor or operator with respect to the ways of understanding them by the patient or his / her family member! It is essential and a priority that what we say is understood exactly for what it means. And if we inquire about the social environment in which the patient lives and the work he does, it will be easier for us to use the most suitable expressions to make him understand exactly his problem, avoiding both underestimating the implications of the disease and enlarging his own infirmity and suffering with the ghosts of the arcane. My dad always said to me: "Remember to speak in "the language of the sick" and not in "the language of the doctors." We must also remember that the sick are not always in the same mood: in the morning they are sometimes disoriented and far from their environment, in the evening they tend to become melancholic. You must use the right tone according to their mood, not our own. Those who cannot speak simply and clearly will hardly know how to communicate and those who cannot communicate will hardly reach the purpose of making people understand what they know.

At the end of these reflections on "health" aesthetics, the considerations made by the art critic Fernando Rigon on the occasion of a banquet come to mind of our Italian Academy of Cuisine, on synaesthesia, or on the way of preparing or tasting a dish using all our senses: sight, smell, taste, hearing and touch. In patient care and in the process of seeking his well-being, we must take into account that every patient has a multi-sensory perception of his condition. For this reason, if we want our treatments to be more effective, we must create beautiful, colorful and illuminated environments that satisfy the view; avoid unnecessary and annoying noise in the hearing; avoid bad smells by spreading pleasant aromas in the rooms; offer palatable foods that tickle the taste despite an unfriendly diet; provide armchairs and beds that are pleasant to the touch, that is, welcoming and clean. Sometimes it takes so little! But that little must be thought of, wanted, built, and managed day by day. Things don't happen, you have to make them happen.

The water of life

IN THE BEGINNING there was fire. Volcanos and craters erupted with a shapeless and incandescent magma that retained part of the energy that feeds the stars. Then, in the progressive condensation of the elements, a type of molecule made of hydrogen and oxygen appeared. The new element, on the one hand had the ability to cool the earth's magma consolidating it, adding more layers, then evaporating rapidly generating the prodrome of a breathable atmosphere. That new element, which irreversibly conditioned the evolution of plant Earth and created the primordial soup in which the germs of plant and animal life would develop, was water. The original liquid element soon became confused with billions of molecules present on the earth's surface to form a high sodium and chlorine content solution that we know today with the name of sea water. And so, in the beginning it was the primordial soup that became the oceans. For this reason, perhaps in the bible and in various ancient cosmogonic theories, we speak of the waters that submerge the lands and the lands that emerge from the waters. And that is why we often talk about the water of life today.

In the great book *"From Fish to Philosopher,"* published in 1956 by the American physiologist Homer William Smith, he proposed an interesting evolutionary theory which suggests each person can be what the kidney allows them to be. But what is the function of the kidney? The kidneys are a complex system of cells, vessels and conduits that has a primary function of purification, or rather the elimination of waste created within our body by the processes of metabolism. Of course, the kidneys also have many other important functions, such as the production of hormones that regulate blood pressure, bone metabolism, and the exchange of red blood cells in the marrow. For the purpose of this story however, we will focus attention on their fundamental regulatory function of the hydro saline and acid-base.

In 1978, Claude Bernard, a French physiologist and great supporter of "Scientific Method" in medicine, wrote an important treatise *Leçons sur les phénomènes de la vie communs aux animaux et aux végétaux* which stigmatized the importance of the balance and constancy of the internal milieu or the "internal medium" which translates roughly to the aqueous component of our body comprising nearly 75% of the body volume of an infant and 60% in an adult. It is the constancy of the "internal medium" that allows us to live.

Claude Bernard wrote: "Although the living body needs a surrounding environment, it is nevertheless relatively independent of it. This independence that the organism has from the external environment derives from the fact that, in the living being, the tissues are isolated from direct external influences and protected from a true internal environment, made up, in particular, of the fluids circulating in the body. The constancy of the internal medium is the condition for free and independent life: the mechanism that makes this possible is the one that ensures the maintenance, in the internal environment, of all the conditions necessary for the life of the organs. The constancy of the environment presupposes a perfection of the organism such that external variations are compensated and kept in balance at all times. Consequently, far from being indifferent to the outside world, the superior animals are in close relationship with it, so that their balance results from a continuous and delicate compensation with a very sensitive balance."

The balance of the water, salts, acids and metal concentrations in our body (called "homeostasis") is maintained within narrow parameters, beyond which serious pathological disorders can appear and vital processes stop. Just think that a variation of about 2 mg/L in the concentration of potassium can give rise to serious cardiac arrhythmias or paralysis; infinitesimal changes in pH (logarithm of the concentration of hydrogen ions) or in calcium can generate convulsions, cardiac arrest and immediate death. But how is it possible that our body knows how to regulate the emission (or rather conservation) of the right amount of body water both when we drink several mugs of beer at the Octoberfest, and when we spend whole days in the desert? How is it possible that the salts are not dispersed or accumulated making the preservation of the "internal medium" difficult if not impossible? The protagonist of maintaining this delicate balance is the kidney which, through metabolic processes of filtration, reabsorption, handling of solutes and control of the elimination of water, preserves the internal milieu always in the same way. Is this why human kidneys are definitely the most complex on the evolutionary scale of animal species. Can the modern philosopher really enunciate his theories thanks to the evolution of his kidneys?

The first forms of animal life developed in the primordial broth of the oceans, which covered most, if not all, of the globe. These single-celled creatures had walls that were easily traversed by ocean convective flows thanks to which the beneficial aqueous solution of genesis brought nourishment to them and dragged away the metabolic by-products: a sort of network balloons in which the vital cytoplasmic solution was renewed continuously. With the evolution of the species, multicellular organisms and progressively more complex forms of life developed up to the fish in which a series of apparatuses, such as the digestive, neural and muscular, are contained in a chitinous envelope made of skin and scales that prevented their exposure and dispersion in the "external medium." The metabolic exchange on the other hand, thanks to a mechanism halfway between that of single-celled beings and that of the most advanced species, is ensured by an internal aqueous flow, and the necessary oxygen for breathing is recovered, through the gills, directly from the water. The great evolutionary leap was represented by amphibians and then, in succession, by reptiles and mammals. All these species had to adapt their biological systems to the inhospitable and arid terrestrial crust. And here the miracle was accomplished by highly evolved organs such as the kidneys, whose function is, in the end, to maintain within the terrestrial organism, and therefore also of man, a small fraction of what was there primordial ocean. Our organism, made up mostly of water and salt, is nothing more than a set of cells that live, as in the beginning, in an internal ocean, the internal milieu. Our kidneys and their purification processes filter a quantity of blood equal to 180 liters every day, regenerating the aqueous component which represents about 65%. Waste, exogenous toxins and metabolic products are filtered, concentrated and eliminated in about one liter of urine. To keep the water at the desired levels in our body, it must be spared, in case of dehydration, and eliminated in case of accumulation, a task performed very well by healthy kidneys. But, in the presence of specific pathologies, the water essential to life can become a poison for the human organism. Just think about a patient suffering from kidney failure who is no longer able to urinate. For these patients, excessive intake of fluids with the diet, can lead to pulmonary edema with water transudation in the lungs. This is why modern medicine has shown a particular interest in research aimed at artificially reproducing the regeneration of plasma water that the healthy kidney already performs spontaneously and seamlessly.

The result is that since the mid-twentieth century we have had an artificial kidney, a hemodialysis technique that allows us to filter the blood and remove metabolic waste and excess water. But each dialysis session involves a consumption of more than 100 liters of ultra-pure water. If we calculate that in Italy about 80,000 patients perform dialysis three times a week, we realize that the water consumption for this therapy is enormous: over one billion liters per year. It is therefore essential to move towards more sustainable kidney replacement therapies. The wearable artificial kidney that we are experiencing at the IRRIV in Vicenza responds to this need and also allows the patient good mobility. However, while the electronics are somewhat easy to miniaturize, the hydraulic circuit is practically incompressible like the fluids circulating in it and therefore the regeneration process is a fundamental step in the development of new systems.

Filtration and water purification systems using filters and adsorbent beds are also of fundamental importance in the industrial world. Recent episodes of contamination of water reservoirs by improperly controlled industrial discharges (pollution by PFAs and PFOA, for example) have produced great interest in the study of new purification systems. Furthermore, the Earth - which observed from space appears blue due to the color of the oceans, lakes and rivers that populate its surface - is now suffering from the considerable quantities of CO_2 responsible for heating the planet and the consequent desertification of vast regions of the globe. The conservation of water, our "blue gold," is fundamental for the survival of the human species since it is a precious component of our diet — a real food. Since ancient times, it was known that rainwater or distilled water were not particularly palatable, while water containing essential salts and metals had a more pleasant taste. For this reason, and according to tradition, water stored in silver jugs acquired a superior flavor and pleasant taste. Today there is a wide variety of waters rich in salts and minerals available to us. We can choose from ferrous or sulfurous water for dietary needs, water with a high calcium for osteoporotic patients, low sodium/calcium/minerals for patients suffering from edema or stones. Although the quality of the drinking water supply guaranteed by our aqueducts is extraordinarily high, the consumption of mineral water is really high and not always justified. Obviously there is justification where purity and microbiologic quality are in question. Great efforts to make unhealthy waters drinkable or to desalinate marsh or even marine waters have been successful today thanks to new filtration technologies and reverse osmosis. This also made it possible to create new oases and settlements in environments that are hostile or naturally precluded to man. The regeneration process of water from exhausted fluids are of great interest, among other things for a possible space colonization plan. It is unthinkable to transport tons of water to the space shuttles to ensure survival of astronauts or future remote settlements. The importance of water for human life is not less than that of air we breathe, and given the high consumption and critical nature to sustain life, there is a real danger of critical situations of deficiency. The progressive desertification of large areas on the planet is a concrete and present danger. How long will our ecosystem be able to withstand different assaults that undermine the entire life cycle?

We must make new generations aware of the good that water represents so they become protagonists in maintaining the system in equilibrium. It wouldn't be a bad idea if young people understood the history and culture of water over the millennia and impact on various civilizations. We could start from the ancient one of the Egyptians that experienced flood of the Nile which was the center and engine of their economy and livelihood, not unlike the Mesopotamian people whose lands were made fertile by the irrigations provided by the Tigris and Euphrates rivers. We also shouldn't forget the Roman Empire. Their unparalleled scientific knowledge and technical expertise in construction of aqueducts are testified by the vestiges of these extraordinary works scattered throughout Europe and the Mediterranean area. It should also be explained to young people that water is so important for life, that it has also always been considered sacred and a source of symbols and rites in all religions. It is a symbol of purification in the baptismal rite of Christians because as Tertullian says. "water was the first seat of the divine spirit which preferred it to all other elements...It was the water that first had the task of generating living creatures." In the four Vedas of the Hindu world, water is described as the incarnation of God and protector of the earth and environment. Even for the shamanic tradition of Native American tribes, water contained the Great Spirit, so much that invoking rain was equivalent to invoking the Great Spirit. For Australian Aborigines, the rain wizard was the most important character of their villages. I have personally been able to see for myself how precious water is for its real and symbolic value, it has been in the great African continent where many ceremonies of everyday life, from wedding ceremonies to the tribal chief coronations, foresee the sprinkling of water on the earth as a symbol of life and prosperity.

One day a friend of mine, Dr. Parise, came into my office and spoke about an association called Madrugada which was based in Verona. It had been bringing aid and work to the remote area of Guinea Bissau for over 15 years. Dr Parise had built a small hospital and asked if would help them organize a dialysis center. He told me "in Guinea there are several cases of kidney failure and chronically renal patients need to emigrate to Portugal or Morocco if they can afford it. Otherwise, they are destined to die without assistance."

"Listen," I told him,"The problem of the chronically ill doesn't have an easy solution, even here, but I can help you solve the acute problem. Patients who due to diarrhea, an insect bite or snake bite have transient kidney damage that can often be treated with a few dialysis sessions. We can definitely organize this."

The following month, Dr Parise arrived with a delegation of Guinean friends, including the country ambassador. We organized a meeting with the management of my hospital and someone from the Region so that we could count on institutional coverage. Our approach to dealing with problems involves putting them on the table and starting a collegial dialogue that includes not just doctors, but also engineers, pharmacists, biologists and economists. Occasionally Fabio, our sociologist also joins in contributing to the socio-economic aspects of the project. To develop a dialysis center in Guinea Bissau, we would need equipment, but also needed to be sure that the electricity grid was reliable. We needed filters and bloodlines, but we also needed to be sure that the staff would be well trained. This is why I included in my projects, an intensive training internship in Vicenza for doctors and nurses from that country. We also ensured collaboration with a small analysis laboratory alongside the African hospital and assured that there was a pharmacy that would be available to support patients at or before the dialysis session, during and after. And yet, above all we needed water! Water that was pure enough to be further filtered by our purification systems. Water that doesn't contain pollutants or bacteria, but also that doesn't contain sediment that can eventually clog filters. Water that has a reserve to provide a constant flow and sufficient for performing multiple treatments without running low.

At that point, Dr. Parise entered with a technician that told us that they had opted for the maintenance of the hydraulic systems of Central Africa and assured me that they had a good well — incredibly — and that they were also digging a backup well. Water would not be a problem! We would still need to ensure the supply of spare equipment parts, an uninterruptible power supply, adequate beds where you could apply scales to follow the weight of the patient during dialysis, filters and disposable circuits for a certain number of mono-use treatments, needles, patches and disinfectants. Above all, we needed a maintenance program for the water production and filtration system. "It will not be easy" I told Dr. Parise, "but we will do it."

A few years have now passed and Guinea Bissau has its small dialysis center with the quality mark of our department. The water that rises from the well discovered near the hospital is now truly the "water of life."

Navigating into profound space

IF THE KIDNEY was undoubtedly the determining element in the passage between marine life and terrestrial life, this fantastic organ could return to the center of the evolution of our species allowing the passage from the life of man on earth to the life of the man in deep space. Of course, we don't know if, and when, we will reach the stars, and the development of an engine that allows these jumps in hyperspace is still science fiction. But the hypothesis is not peregrine since plans are already being drawn up to visit the planets of our solar system and establish colonies of humans there. For that matter, given that our continents are now simple neighborhoods of a global city, why not satisfy the irrepressible desire to widen the boundaries of our knowledge and verify if we Earthlings are the only inhabitants of a small sphere within a universe too big to be deserted? It shouldn't be forgotten that in the future the Earth could be an environment so polluted and depleted of the resources necessary for life that the human race will be forced to imitate the nomadism of primitive populations and emigrate to more livable worlds.

The interest in astronautics, interplanetary flight and interstellar travel has always been alive in me, but it has heightened in recent days following an extraordinary meeting that has to do with my profession as a nephrologist and a health worker. Everything started from an international phone call, disturbed by a loud background hum: "Am I talking to Professor Ronco? Professor Claudio Ronco?" he asked with a strong Eastern European accent. "I am calling you from Moscow and wish to bring to your attention the problem of one of our illustrious patients." He told me that he was a colleague from the Baculiev Clinic, an important cardiac surgery center where I had taught a few times. "The person who asks for your help as an internationally renowned nephrologist is a hero of the Soviet nation." I had a slight uneasiness that perhaps the call was a hoax, but the caller assured me that the phone call had been authorized at the highest levels and tells me that the person who suggested he contact me is an ice hockey fan that remembered my lecture from a few years ago. He had also planted a tree near mine in the clinic garden. All of this convinced me that the call was genuine. He described an 86-year-old diabetic hypertensive patient with some degree of chronic renal failure suddenly aggravated. He was a national hero that was looking for the best clinic and great discretion.

I immediately raised the concern that moving such a critically ill patient could lead to serious complications and that a flight could even be fatal. The Russian colleague continued with persistence and told me that with my consent, the patient would be transported by a private plane to Italy that day.

I obtained the authorization from the General Director of our San Bortolo Hospital in Vicenza and the patient arrived in the early evening from the Verona airport. He suffered from acute kidney dysfunction linked to heart failure and needed dialysis. We began the dialysis treatment that evening and continued it for the following days in which he had an improvement in the contractile function of the heart and stabilization of the diabetes. Within a week, the elderly patient urinated regularly, appeared in a better shape, and was able to eat independently. I relaxed a bit and asked him to tell me about himself. He told me to call him Aleksej Andropovich Leonov. I was speechless! As a bit of a space exploration fan, I understood right away that I was in front of the legendary Leonov, the first man in the world to perform an EVA — that is an Extra-Vehicular Activity, or a walk in space outside the orbiting capsule.

Aleksej told me how dramatic it was for him for his first exit from the spacecraft. Due to an incorrect calculation of the pressures, which had not taken into account the internal hydrostatic gradient with respect to the sidereal vacuum, his suit had swelled to the point of not allowing him to return to the narrow space of the capsule. Aleksej was forced to unscrew a valve and vent oxygen in the void with the risk of losing consciousness and dying of cold in order to return to the capsule! He managed, almost without oxygen to rapidly slash through the very narrow door of the capsule and close it behind him. Old Aleksej, in the presence of his wife and daughter, told me that adventure with pride and energy as if the ailments of age had completely disappeared. The hero, who I had only known in the books from history, was in front of me.

Before he left for Russia, Aleksej gave me a monograph full of photos and drawings dedicated to his long career. After his first adventure, he had participated in other space missions and for twenty five years he had been the director of the aerodrome and spaceport Yuri Gagarin. When he said goodbye, he winked and said to me "Our friend, the hockey player, sends you his regards and assures you that the tree at the Baculiev Clinic will be cared for with the same attention as you have treated this old Bolshevik. He will always be grateful."

The first person who made me think about the relationship between nephrology research and travel to Mars had been a nice space engineer from Reggio Emilia, Tommaso, who lives in Switzerland. He had come to visit me in Vicenza and told me that he was dealing with things that can go wrong in the missions of the European Space Agency. Struck by his intelligence and open-mindedness, I invited him to share his vision on the future of planetary exploration to a diverse but curious audience. The first extraordinary thing he told us was that the travel plan to Mars was already a reality and that the key tool for the success of the mission could be a 3D printer. He explained to us that a three dimensional printer is like a fax, which instead of imprinting the message from the computer remotely in ink on a sheet, prints structures, elements, three dimensional objects with an "ink" derived from the basic materials making up the object themselves. In this way, all the tools and equipment necessary to prepare the bases for the stay of future explorers of Mars, could be built directly on the red planet with 3D printers that use Martian dust as "ink" instead of transporting them from earth.

This is an interesting concept similar to that of Captain Kirk's teleportation on the Enterprise spaceship. But first, I thought, we will have to deal with the crew. Not everyone would be able to face such a long-lasting stay in space and on Martian soil. It would take 500 days just to make the outward journey and then for the return, it would be necessary to have the correct alignment of the planets to make the most of the gravitational slings and the shortest paths. If all goes well, a return trip of this kind can't last for less than 5 years. Furthermore, on Mars, you can't sit on the deckchair enjoying the sun while waiting to leave, nor in the shelter of the spacecraft which being made of metal only partially deflects the cosmic radiation, if not even concentrating it inside. The high energy particles on earth are blocked by the electromagnetic effect of the poles and imprisoned by the "Allen belts." These are not obstructed on Mars and expose the exploration crew to radiation that is a thousand times higher than that of an orbital mission on the spacelab stationed on a Low Earth Orbit (LEO). All this will force you to created ultra-protective shielded suits for astronauts, adequate shields for spacecraft and, on the red planet, underground shelters (perhaps we should call them sub-walls) or brick igloos made with Martian powder from 3D printers. The crew members must therefore be chosen from people who do not present pathologies at the time of departure and above all from those whose genome will guarantee the onset of pathologies in the long term. This will entail eugenic choices with ethical implications that should not be underestimated, also because in such long-lasting missions, the birth of Martian children will not be unlikely, who, for aesthetic and functional aspects, could be different from the terrestrial prototypes.

In fact, we still know very little about the effects of long space explorations on humans. The observations are mostly limited to short orbital flights where the disturbances that occur are mainly those related to some G+ (multiples of the force of gravity) during the take-off phase and to the readjustment to G1 (normal gravity force) upon return. The negative effects of weightlessness for short periods are reduced to disorientation syndromes with dizziness and headache and a vague sensation of swelling linked to the redistribution of body fluids in the upper body: the "puffy face" effect and chicken legs (thin). The damage to the human body resulting from prolonged stationing on an orbiting space laboratory such as that of Peggy Whitson and Jeff Williams which lasted for more than a year — will certainly be more serious and require more in-depth studies. There is an SAS (space adaptation syndrome) which requires the individual to make a great effort to adapt to the conditions of microgravity, this causes a progressive demineralization of the skeleton and a deconditioning of the muscular system. For now, we try to remedy this with radial constriction suits simulating the earth's gravity and with systematic isometric gymnastic exercises. The entire clinical picture of probable long-term disturbances in space seems particularly interesting for a nephrologist. The loss of calcium salts from the bone found in the urine, together with reduced urine output due to lower water intake, sweating, reduced air humidity and altered hormonal conditions, will favor the formation of kidney stones. An important problem which could be aggravated by urinary tract infections caused by incomplete emptying of the bladder in the absence of gravity. To prevent the formation of stones, it will be necessary to study an adequate diet and to foresee the use of some supplements such as citrate and ascorbic acid — the same ones that allowed exploration of the terrestrial oceans eliminating scurvy from the frequent pathologies of seafarers.

In short, the overall clinical picture will have to be addressed by nephrology research. Kidney cells are very rich in mitochondria, the small bodies filled with nucleic acids that supply energy to tissues and organs. Since they are the first to be damaged by oxidative stress phenomena that would transform renal tissue into a dysfunctional fibrous mass, it will be necessary to prepare an artificial renal support for space explorers, which could consist of a wearable and compatible miniaturized dialysis system compatible with the protective suit. But we could also be forced to focus on regenerative medicine, which, to tell the truth works better in less sophisticated animal species: think, for example, of the regeneration of the claws of crabs and the tails of lizards. In humans, the high specialization of organs and tissues makes spontaneous regeneration almost impossible. An external approach could then be used using frozen stem cells. Some stem cells, once thawed, can be induced with appropriate stimuli, to multiply and specialize to become the cells that make up specific tissues. This has already been done for skin and bone tissue. These cells called mesenchymal stromal cells are present in embryonic blood and in large quantities in the umbilical cord and have a special tropism for damaged and inflamed areas and could help with repair and regeneration of damaged tissue. Although it seems obvious that they could be damaged by the same insult that damaged the tissues they are supposed to repair. Finally, some approaches are being studied to treat kidney damage occurring in space crews.

Although this may seem like science fiction, there is already an advanced study with encouraging results in an animal kidney, that removed the cellular part while maintaining the architecture of the vessels and the fibrous skeleton in which then cells could be injected to colonize the organ and develop advanced anato-functional structures. Another would even provide for the printing of real human tissues and organs with 3D machines based on bio-inks (I.e., mixtures of amino acids, nucleic acids and pre-formed cells). In short, starting from the mission to Mars, the crews sent to space will have to rely on advanced techniques of reparative and regenerative medicine. The rudiments of medicine, such as those initially provided to today's astronauts then will be insufficient. Communications between Earth and deep spaceships will come with delays that won't be sufficient to allow corrective actions or interventions in real time. We will therefore need to have an on-board doctor and the spacecraft will need to be equipped for emergencies such as the "sick-bay" of the Starship Enterprise. Curious how science fiction once again precedes science. Thinking back to Leonov's story, and reading the notes that my friend Tommaso occasionally sends me from the ESA headquarters, makes me want to think about paraphrasing a consideration written by Christopher Columbus while navigating the new world; "and space will bring to every man new hopes as the night brings dreams."

Dear Mars, wait for us. We are coming.

Carpediem

"CARPE DIEM, quam minimum credula postero" (Seize the present; trust tomorrow e'en as little as you may), said Horace in his odes and so this must be the thought of a doctor who faces an emergency in a difficult patient. There is no time to waste and you must act as if there is no tomorrow, because your patient's tomorrow depends on what you do at this precise moment. It's half past six in the evening and with Alessandra, my trusted colleague and friend, we are reviewing a report for her thesis. It is 1979, we have developed a new therapy for acute renal failure to be applied in particular for critically ill patients. A sort of autonomous artificial kidney that works by connecting it directly to the patient's circulation. For some time now, our new technologies have been proposed as a point of reference and the research and development teams of many companies have paid attention to our studies and projects. Alessandra's thesis deals precisely with these innovative technologies developed in our department. The department chief abruptly entered the narrow room of our "on call" office, and tells us that there is an urgency in pediatric surgery. We have to run. I put up a little resistance as I don't have the best relationship with the chief of that department, but my boss doesn't hear us. We arrive breathless and between cables and monitors we glimpse at small bundle in a cradle with a large visible scar on the chest and abdomen.

"This is a little boy who has operated on for a serious heart malformation - says Sandro, the cardiac surgeon — "and he has not urinated for five hours. We had to do something quickly. The traditional dialysis, peritoneal dialysis, that we perform by adding liquid to the abdomen could not be done because of the large scar making it impractical. I could feel the tension rise. Alessandra looked at me with questions as we sat down to look at the exams. The soft lights of the pediatric ICU and the hum of the equipment transported us to a parallel world — muffled, almost surreal. Sandro had been trained in France by Professor Aubert and was considered one of the best pediatric cardiac surgeons in Italy and perhaps in Europe. I had no doubts regarding the surgery, but the baby's small kidneys were gravely compromised. I thought about it, and then proposed an extreme attempt. We had just developed a mini filter for laboratory experiments that allowed us to simulate extracorporeal circulations at low volumes. This is exactly what it would take for our little Francesco, who would otherwise die. The treatment had never been performed on patients, but since even the surly department chief was also in agreement we decided to go ahead. I had to connect that small filter that I had designed for experimental studies with an artery and a vein of the child. It would then be Francesco's own heart, newly repaired, that would then work to pump the blood through the circuit. We sterilized the materials and prepared the circuit and applied the filter. Incredibly the system worked! The filter eliminates the "waste" that normally would be cleared by the kidneys as urine. After four days of treatment, Francesco improved, and his kidneys recovered. We won. Sandro embraced me warmly, while even the department chief shook my hand. Finally, Alessandra and I could take a break and we got a pizza to eat in the resident doctor's office room. We looked at the data for her thesis and decided to also include the case of little Francesco.

My boss told the president of the hospital that we had performed a procedure that had never been done before. The hospital involved the local papers. We had to go back and slowly re-evaluate the data and document what we did. We wrote up the protocol and communicated to the world.

After we had treated three other neonates with similar conditions, we gathered the consent of the international community and published in the scientific journal, Kidney International. The article attracted the attention of an American company which offered to develop the device and produce it on an industrial scale. I entrusted the direction of the project to my engineer friend Luciano, with whom I had developed the prototypes that we had used. Shortly afterwards, I was called to illustrate and apply my method of pediatric dialysis in various American universities.

Thirty years had passed since I had first treated Francesco, and although adult dialysis technologies had made considerable progress, this had not been the case for dialytic treatments for children. There are relatively few cases of acute pediatric renal failure and very little interest from industry to develop treatments, much less to do research in this area.

Pediatricians whose skills are often limited, attempt to transfer adult dialysis technologies to the infant, but adaption is not always particularly effective, particularly in the complex therapies for infants. It would be like trying to adapt a wrench to fix a clock. The pathology that affects children is in fact considered "orphaned" since even our arterio-venous small 30-year filter had pretty much run its course. It would take new and modern solutions.

I started looking for a company between America and Japan that would agree to develop the project for miniaturized dialysis for the newborn. There was no commercial interest and the doors remained closed. After many years of waiting, I decided to propose to my friend Luciano that we collaborate on a new project that could be developed in Italy between Vicenza and Mirandola. Mirandola was already home to most of the new technologies for dialytic therapies. It was here that I found the solution to tackle the problem of a dialytic solution specifically adapted to infants and small children.

When I told Luciano about my idea, he immediately said "I'm in," but also asked that we involve Domenico, a friend of his and an engineer from a nearby company. He was a person with an enormous heart and was willing to help even from the garage at his house.

After I had returned from a meeting in Chicago, I found the first sketches of what would be our future dialysis machine for neonates. Luciano and Domenico produced designs that were not typical "professional designs, but they captured the essence of the project and the search began for the components to design the first prototype. Our institute, IRRIV, was initially located in a single room and crammed with students, post-graduates and researcher that began to work decisively with analyses, calculations and tests to support my project.

A big help came from a dear old friend whose chair was put on display in the room in front of the dean at the University of Padua, Galileo Galilei. The great scientist was obsessed with the dimensional question and, in having described the law of the square/cube, he had dedicated long observations to the infinitely large with the telescope and to the infinitely small with the microscope of his invention. He understood why dinosaurs could not run and why larger birds have more difficulty with flight — in essence, he grasped the capacity to understand the size factor. After him, many other scientists grappled with enigmatic problems of size, up to Richard Feynman, who won the Nobel prize for physics and quantum cosmology and that madman Eric Drexler, pioneer of nanotechnologies. Reading Galileo I understand that I must not simply shrink the adult dialysis machine, but rather confront myself with the laws of physics and invent a completely new operating system. To find the funding that would allow us to quickly proceed, I decided to create a solidarity mechanism fueled by a series of show-events promoted by voluntary associations, primarily by the "Friends of the Kidney" of Vicenza and by the Association of Craftsmen; a concert by the police academy (Arma dei Carabinieri), the Orfei Circus; Ciccio and his band; and the commedie of Goldoni.

The events accompanied the various stages of the project until in 2008 we arrived at the first working prototype. Sandro, the world-renowned heart surgeon, with whom we had worked together for the first dialysis treatment, gave a speech in Vicenza and said, "with this machine, we will cure many cases that previously were untreatable." CARPEDIEM will make a qualitative leap forward in neonatal and pediatric care." In the end, I decided to call our machine **CARPEDIEM**, an acronym that stands for *Cardio Renal Pediatric Dialysis Emergency Machine*, but also alludes to the need to "seize the moment," that moment between life and death that can really make the difference for a newborn baby with severe cardio-renal problems. The authorities participated in the press conference, although I wasn't sure they understood the true meaning of the invention and the consensus that surrounded our work and allowed us to proceed at a record pace. The construction of the new Renal Research Institute was also proceeding quickly, and our project seemed to galvanize the Vicenza community and beyond. In the laboratory we continued to test our equipment under conditions of maximum stress. We tried with saline solutions, then with bovine blood and finally with blood from human donors. Much of that blood comes actually from our own research staff, as well as my own, compensated with some high-quality salami sandwiches. Domenico continued to work largely on his own without involving his company, while Luciano and his company produced the disposable plastic circuits to try and produce products with the best compatibility possible between the materials and patient blood. We worked tirelessly occupying all the free time possible between rounds, consultations and visits.

In the meantime, I had become the chief of the department and I had to manage many other responsibilities. This didn't always allow me to spend as much time as I had wanted (I really wanted to devote myself body and soul to the project), but I also had the strong solidarity and commitment of the entire team. When it was time to finally choose the color, we decided on a warm pink-red-orange, the color of the many mornings dawn that we have seen from our laboratory after sleepless nights of work, the color of sunrise, the color of life that is renewed.

The colleagues I meet at pediatric conferences do not understand how an adult nephrologist came to deal with the problems of infants and the quiet murmur of envious and malevolent whispers make me realize that the problem is far from resolved. True friends however know the competence, quality and passion of our team and have no doubts that something good will come out of so many efforts. Finally on July 13, 2013, after five years of tests and checks, the machine — financed entirely by benefactors and volunteers, was approved for human use by the Ministry. There was no time even for a celebration however to celebrate this milestone because on August 26, while I was abroad for a conference, I received a phone call from Alessandra informing me of a very serious case of a newborn baby that had suffered trauma during birth. From that moment, the story of Lisa began with the machine on which her life depended (see the entire story told in the book *CARPEDIEM*, IngramSpark, USA).

The hair-thin cannula (the tiny tube that gets inserted into the baby's blood vessel to connect the machine) had never been used before. It had been too small for the classic adult machines. The blood volumes in the circuit are very low (how much of the baby's blood is needed to circulate outside the body for the machine during treatment). There were no guidelines. We had to write history at that moment.

I contacted an American colleague at Cincinnati Children's hospital via SMS and he texted back that we would probably go nowhere. After a week of 24 hours a day sustained treatments, the American colleagues told us they couldn't believe what we were doing was possible. At the first signs of improvement, after CARPEDIEM continued to purify Lisa's blood for days, our friends at Cincinnati told us it was a miracle At the end of the fourth week of treatment, and after days and nights of apprehensions, enthusiasms, fear, moments of panic, partial successes, we were finally able to extubate (take out the breathing tube) the girl from the mechanical respirator and remove the artificial kidney: Lisa was able to breathe freely and urinate independently. The severe syndrome has been overcome and the disease was triumphantly defeated. The little girl returned to life thanks to our machine. Stuart Goldstein from the Cincinnati pediatric hospital declared "This will change medicine for the newborns. Now we want CARPEDIEM in America and we will do everything to make the little miracle of Vicenza cross the ocean." It is a recognition of a victory that returns to us after so much work, opposition and bitterness. It was one step on a long path. After a glass of prosecco with my team of researchers, we returned together towards our Institute because there was still so much work to do. But we also know that pediatric renal failure would never be again considered an orphan disease. Children now had CARPEDIEM.

The story of Gio' — born and born again

WHAT SHOULD THE life of a thirty-year old young man be like? Effervescent, full of hope, joyful, carefree, enthusiastic, exciting, incredible? Giovanni Fattori's life was all of this. He was born to a bourgeois family. He had a diploma in accounting, but knew he would never be an accountant. He had discovered the world of fashion very early and already at 31 he was leading a small successful company in a town in the upper Vicenza area that supplied leather to Prada, Gucci and other luxury brands. He had worked hard and traveled like crazy, but it had been worth it and, still young, he had a discreet nest egg aside with which he could afford a comfortable life.

Two years earlier he had met a sweet Slovenian girl named Lara, who worked as a secretary next to his company. The two had immediately liked each other. They began dating and were married within a few months. A short time later, Andrea was born and brought further happiness to the family. Lara had quit work, and managed the accounts of Giovanni's company by computer from home. The demand for products from Giovanni's company far exceed their production capacity. Everything was going well, work proceeded, and they had built a small villa on the hills of Vicenza. Giovanni traveled a lot and allowed himself only a few amusements. They took a couple of holidays by the sea or in the mountains and occasionally went to visit his parents who always took advantage of being able to spoil their grandson. Sometimes they went to Cipriani in Venice, happy to be able to afford the luxury of a motorboat, a refined dinner and a quick trip to the casino. Money seemed to come in avalanches and he had the feeling of being on a carousel destined to turn endlessly.

Giovanni felt full of energy and had a strong desire to work, but occasionally he suffered from stomach acid and felt a little dizzy. These symptoms didn't seem too serious and were passed off to stress. Lara also saw these things every now and then, but after all, it didn't seem so strange when working sixteen hours a day and traveling the world like a top. She also thought that her husband had no reason to worry. That spring, they were taking three days of vacation to ski In Val Badia. Already on the first day however Giovanni suffered a few degrees of fever and didn't leave the room. Lara, accustomed to her husband's natural exuberance was a little worried, now seeing him sweaty and weak. When they returned home, they decided to put the experience past them and attribute it to a small influence. Giovanni however continued to take antacids and increasingly used headache medicine. He now had a continuous pounding headache that that rarely ceased. Once again, he attributed these ailments to overwork and stress.

In May, Giovanni's attention was monopolized by the arrival of his latest purchase: a brand new Ferrari 328 GTs. He had to do a bit of waiting because, you know, Ferrari won't sell you a car right away, even if you pay in cash. Giovanni however had provided the Maranello Company (Ferrari) with leather for the seats of a special edition reserved for the Arab Emirates with crazy customizations. For this reason, the waiting times were less biblical than normal. In the summer they went to Castiglioncello and bought a Riva yacht used by a Tuscan entrepreneur. On that occasion, he also combined the purchase with that of a small estate in Chianti where the entrepreneur had produced excellent wine as a hobby. It seemed there were no limits to the things that Giovanni and Lara could desire and have.

Giovanni's company was now going on without the need of a lot of guidance. Production and sales ran well. It was a good economic time for Italy. Giovanni had found himself at the right place, at the right time, in the middle of the northeastern economic boom. Everything seemed to be going well. Life flowed calmly in the Fattori house. Little Andrea was growing day by day. The grandparents helped the young couple by occasionally keeping the little one and filling those educational gaps that, in their opinion, the couple had left out of Andrea's life. Lara smiled at the grandparents who spoiled him, while Giovanni continued to run like crazy: business trips by train and plane, Ferrari trips, speedboat rides. Nothing forewarned the fate that would soon manifest for them.

Giovanni for some time had lost some energy. He started going regularly to a gym to take advantage of the moments of pause between flights to the Middle East to negotiate new supplies or other flights to Brazil to select lots of skins. He thought that exercise would help him relieve tension and do him good. He also had met a group of young men, more or less his age, who at the beginning of summer had put together a five-a-side soccer team for an amateur tournament. They played the first game on the first Saturday of April. At half-time Giovanni's team was leading by 2-0 and there was an excited air in the locker room. Giovanni however collapsed and fell into unconsciousness on the locker room bench after drinking half a glass of tea. His teammates tried to revive him and immediately called the emergency number. Giovanni regained consciousness when he heard the wail of the ambulance siren and tried to pass off the incident due to the heavy lunchtime meal. His friends however convinced him to get things checked out at the nearby Vicenza hospital as the emergency workers arrived.

It was a beautiful spring day. The scent of the blossoms

from the park had invaded the doctor's study room where I was working on a report for the American Congress of Artificial Organs while I was on duty. The buzzer rang and I could see the emergency room number. I rushed down the stairs and reached the emergency room. "Doctor, we have a thirty-five year old man with a syncopal episode and ongoing hypertensive crisis. We have no news of his past-history." Meanwhile, I tried to control the sky-high blood pressure and stabilize the patient. I then turned towards him and asked him his name. "Giovanni Fattori, but call me Gio' doctor."

"Well, Gio', have you had any other episodes like this? Have you had any major illnesses? Are you taking any medication?"

"No, no particular disease that I remember and I don't take any medicines except painkillers for a recurring headache I have had for years. The only thing is that I make a lot of urine, especially at night, but I think it's normal since I drink a lot in the evening." He seemed both scared and a little angry.

"Alright," I said, "Now let's lower the pressure and then wait for the results of the urgent tests," I tell him, trying to calm him down and put him at ease, "but have you ever had high blood pressure Gio?"

He replied, "I've never measured it in my life. I have a family and a company to run and I can't afford to feel bad."

We gave him an injection and waited for a progressive reduction in pressure that started to drop from 220/150, but not by much. We applied monitoring. Finally the pressure started to trend towards acceptable values only after the second injection. The results of the first exam arrived and, in the meantime, his wife also arrived. "Ma'am, stay close to Gio" and consider that he needs to stay calm and rested. For today we will continue to monitor his pressure and stabilize him. I'll take him up to the ward to keep him under observation. I'll put you in a room for two and so, if you want, you can also stay the night."

I see their faces partly reassured by the certainty of being followed and partly worried by the lack of an adequate explanation. I don't feel like giving any further explanation that evening, even though I understand that we are facing a serious situation and I will have to make further checks, an ultrasound and repeat the exams. Tonight, I am on watch, so we can continue the care. I need to get a little familiar with them. I need them to trust and have faith. Gio' is the classic entrepreneur from the Italian northeast who seems capable of breaking the mountains and not stopping in front of anything. I have a fear however that this time he will have to stop, and it won't be easy to explain it or make him accept it.

Gio' had spent an agitated night and was unable to stay confined to the hospital room. Lara had rested a little, always kept her eyes down and seemed to not want to ask questions, much less receive answers. I had gone to them every two hours for a series of checks and to chat a bit in order to get to know them better and make myself known. Now we know enough about each other. We have almost the same age and quite similar ideas, expectations and dreams. I had Gio' tell of his bravado about the Ferrari, the rides on the motorboat and I learned about leather and tanning in general. I went to the kitchen to retrieve two coffees and a little warm milk and return to the room after viewing the ultrasound that had been done earlier urgently. It is one of those moments that I would like to escape from that cage of suffering found in the hospital. Not only because after twenty-four hours of service that I am exhausted, but because I have to deliver news that will be life-shattering to this poor young couple.

I begin. "Gio', Lara, I don't have a better way to tell you, and so I will get to the point like an old friend would do. Your hypertension Gio' seems to be a malignant form and it was not only yesterday that it has been causing you harm. Frequent headaches are a sign of the disease and all the vessels in your body are suffering. Kidney damage was caused by hypertension and the medications you took for headache. Your kidneys work — "more or less" at about 10% of normal. We are faced with irreversible and progressive damage. From here, we can't go back, and we cannot heal." I lower my head and remain silent as their faces turn white and they are left without words. I know they are wondering if they should believe this young doctor who just told them their world is collapsing. Is it possible that there is someone who knows more? Is it possible that with money and knowledge that one can't find adequate care? Maybe in America? They would like to know more, they would like to be able to change the course of things, they would like to be in another reality. I try to explain to them that there are therapies that perhaps, in the future, will allow Gio' a normal life. But this will take time and care. I also try to explain that "America" is actually here in Italy where we know how to treat and assist kidney patients better than any other country in the world. "But doctor, if the disease can't be cured and it's progressive, are you trying to say that my kidneys are completely destroyed? They will never work again? How will I live with this?"

"Listen Gio', you are a businessman, a practical and strong man. I don't want to hide the truth. You will live and perhaps live well, but you will need to have a particular treatment with an artificial kidney — dialysis."

"Dialysis? The cleansing of the blood? Every two days? What kind of life would that be? And for all my life?"

"I hope not for always, but for the moment, yes. We will try to find a solution that is acceptable and wait for the only thing that can restore normalcy — a kidney transplant." I don't know if there is right way to say such a thing. Some want to know the details of the disease, others — just deny the existence of the problem. Some don't understand, others pretend not to understand and have the same story repeated once, twice, ten times. There is no painless way to give a person the news of the storm that is about to fall on their life. The problem I face every time I have to give this information is to guess the right way to make the patient and their family feel my closeness and hope to make them suffer as little as possible. But however, we put it, the storm will eventually come.

After less than a week since Gio' and Lara arrived in our department, we really began to know each other. I learned to take the angry and pissed-off entrepreneur with the world that had been heading in the right direction and make him understand that I was doing my best to make him feel good. He was very impressed by the fact that I had just returned from the United States. In the evening, we often found ourselves chatting in the room that now also Lara had moved into. She brought him food — since hospital food is terrible. She bought him a television because the one in the room was small and an armchair because the one in the hospital didn't seem comfortable enough for her husband. In short, she tried to provide Gio' with a sense of wellbeing that was ensured by small domestic comforts. Now, the moment has arrived to explain how dialysis works for the day that is drawing nearer. This moment isn't easy. I maintain a little distance and sit at the foot of the bed and start talking about my first day in the dialysis ward as a young specialist. I was deathly afraid, also because I was worried the nurses would ask me questions that I wouldn't know how to answer. I was also afraid that patients would read uncertainty and hesitation in my eyes and feel they were entrusted to unsafe hands.

Gio' smiled at my confession of weakness and felt almost obliged to cheer me up. As a good entrepreneur, he would also like to reorganize pieces of my past life. I let him speak, then gently brought the discussion back to where I wanted it to go. "Gio', your kidneys have suffered damage that is beyond repair. We can provide some medication, but we can't repair what is irreparably damage. We must replace their function and that is what we do with the artificial kidney. Don't worry though — my knowledge has improved a lot since my first time in the dialysis ward. Now you can trust me. Lara and I will lead you by the hand in your new life. Believe me, it's worse to talk about it than actually undergo dialysis!"

Giovanni goes from a state of bewilderment to a sort of aggression, which is fear, irrationality. He had a need to vent. I began to calmly explain to him how the blood was washed by way of filters that we use for extracorporeal dialysis and how the machines work. But while I see his face darkening with the prospect of spending three days a week in the hospital, I also gain his interest by presenting new possibilities. "See Gio', years ago, people simply died of your illness. Then, in the years shortly after the discovery of dialysis, there were not enough machines for everyone, and we had to choose who could live and who was destined for a different fate. Subsequently, we managed to reduce the dialysis time from 12 to 4 hours per session, with maximum comfort — including television, computer and internet connection during the session. Nevertheless, patients must still come to the hospital three times a week. But for you, once we have passed this first period in which we will do some session with a cannula to be inserted in the jugular vein, I see the possibility to do home hemodialysis. In collaboration with an American company that has just developed equipment for a treatment called peritoneal dialysis. In essence, instead of extracting the blood and cleaning it outside the body, we apply a catheter to your abdomen and insert clean liquid in cycles. When the liquid adsorbs the waste, we discharge — or remove it from your abdomen, and then add new fresh clean fluid. In the evening, while watching television or snuggling with your wife, you can connect to the treatment machine which will last until seven in the morning. Then you will be completely free during the day.

Gio' looked at me as though in a trance and said "You are a doctor, I understand that I have no choice but to trust, but know that if it isn't as you say, I will throw myself out the window."

I replied, "For the moment, peritoneal dialysis will be your new kidney and you will be well again. Then we will think about the future and find ways to make you move like a champion again."

I walked slowly out and scrolled my hand along the rough walls of the corridor. Like many times before, I feel overwhelmed by the burden of illness of the people that rely on me. It is too big to explain and worse to bear. At that moment, Giuliano, our head nurse came to me and said with a beaming smile — "Doctor, my first daughter Anna was born!" And so, once again between joy and sorrow, between drama and an extraordinary event, I continue my life as a doctor giving the maximum of my knowledge and by studies so that the tragedy of Gio' becomes a potential rebirth.

It was Christmas Eve and Gio' and Lara came to see me. Gio' had been on home peritoneal dialysis for about six months. They brought me a basket full of good things and the almond nougat that I love.

"Doctor, you don't know how grateful we are for all that you have done and are doing for us now. On that now distant Spring day when we met and you told me about my future, I wanted to kill you. I wasn't ready, but you found the right way to make us understand and made me feel I was cared for. You didn't just heal me; you took care of us like we were your relatives. When you told me, it was more difficult to talk about dialysis than to actually do it, I didn't believe you. But now, I am here to tell you that you were right and to thank you. I was in New York, Dubai and Buenos Aires for work and was able to do dialysis in a hotel where you had helped me find the machine, the materials and bags. Do you know, I even went on a four-day sailing trip! I seem to be reborn, my strength has returned and pressure has settled. You are a magician. I hope the next step is transplantation, but in the meantime, I want my company to participate in some

way in your commitment by supporting your researchers. I decided to make funds available for a scholarship for a young graduate student, and one of these evenings I will invite you to dinner for a nice barbecue. I will keep to my diet and drink less, but I have learned the ritual of ice (dialysis patients can calm their thirst without drinking large quantities of water by keeping an ice cube in their mouth) and that of food mindfulness. I want to get my transplant in perfect shape."
"Doctor I won't give up until this is all fixed. Dialysis saved me and I will cry it out to the four winds to help all those who have to start and have the same lingering doubts and fears that I had.

The next months passed with swiss-like precision. Gio's new life allowed him to still take boat trips, business trips, and drives in his Ferrari. Thanks to his positive attitude and optimism, dialysis had become an instrument in his life rather than a hellish impediment.

That Spring, I called Gio' and Lara and told them that Gio's blood pressure had stabilized and there was no reason to further delay being placed on the transplant list. Giovanni and Lara looked at me partially exhausted because again I was turning their lives upside down, just when they had reached a reassuring balance. But once again, they needed to trust and have faith. "It will be what God wants," they say.

Daniele Carretta was a mechanic from a small town in the Vicenza area with his own workshop where he worked with passion and a lot of skill. Whether it was a tractor, car or moped — all engines that had a problem could be fixed by Daniele. But Daniele's real great passion was large motorcycles. Since he wasn't married, he was able to follow every Grand Prix that took place in Italy and often found himself on the paddock of an important race because even the most noble mechanics of competition motorcycle manufacturers willing accepted his advice and sometimes even sought it. The previous week Daniele had been to Mugello and had fulfilled his dream of being able to talk to

Valentino Rossi. The meeting with the champion had set off a spark. He worked vigorously throughout the week and, on Sunday, had decided to give himself a reward for a ride on the Costo road of Asiago with his Kawasaki Ninja. He felt the thrill of the wind on his helmet and leather suit and the fast accelerations on the uphill straights and the controlled tilts on the curves galvanized him. The first part of his "race" was ruined by a bus that had forced him to stay behind it for two hairpin turns. Then he decided at the parking area of a restaurant to return to Cogollo and redo the climb hoping to have better luck and beat his personal best. But between the 3rd and 4th hairpin turn in a curve to the left around and what everyone refers as Monte Rotondo, Daniele had an appointment with his destiny. He encountered another large cylinder motorcycle that had taken the curve too widely and had no possibility to reduce his speed. The two rearview mirrors touched and Daniele flew out of the guard rail and fell two turns lower on the road.

He couldn't feel anything — just the asphalt on his back. He had no pain and was surprised that everyone was around him. The emergency helicopter arrived, and they immediately brought him to the Vicenza hospital. Daniele could hear the doctors speak on the radio alerting of the need for urgent care. He didn't understand what was happening. He slowly fell into an irreversible coma. His spinal cord had been truncated by the accident and the large bleeding that had formed inside the cranial cavity obstructed the passage of blood to the brain by compressing it. Daniele was dying. He could be supported for a few hours with the support of the machine for extracorporeal breathing support, but there was nothing else left to do. The head of the ICU called me on the phone and described the case to me. I understood what he wanted to say. I rushed in and found him talking to Daniele's parents. When I arrived, his mother and father, two very dignified and reserved people looked and recognized me.

"Doctor, we saw you on television last week and I know who you are and what you do. Your colleague explained to me that there is no hope for Daniele and I can only tell her that I will respect my son's wishes. Three months ago, he joined the Italian Organ Donor Association. Of course, we give our consent."

The two elders return to their painful moment and I can only stammer a thank you.

From that moment the observation period begins to decree the brain death of Daniel. He is kept under close observation in case something changes and can ignite a glimmer of hope. But we also know the clinical course of these traumas and the flat electroencephalogram doesn't lie. We report the case to the North Italian Transplant group which organizes the check between Daniele's blood and lymph nodes and checks for a possible match. After a few hours they respond that the liver will go to Pisa, the heart to Padua, one kidney will go to Brescia and the other will remain in Vicenza. The first of the trio of recipients is Mr. Giovanni Fattori (Gio').

Summer nights at the hospital have a silent and muffled atmosphere as if the outside world didn't exist. The silence of the corridors where patients rest is interrupted only by the sporadic alarm of medical. The darkness of the night is illuminated by antiseptic blue lights or by the LEDs of the monitors used to support vital functions. The doctor's room where we wait while on call is spartan and equipped to make operations as quick and effective as possible. Two telephones, a computer, a filing cabinet with the lists of transplant candidates and a cot to rest a little when possible. I have been on duty since morning and the night looked like it would be eventful. The incident on the Costo road triggered the path of donation of poor Daniele's organs. I was waiting for the final confirmation from Milan through the cross match with Gio's blood. I waited impatiently and tapped the linoleum flooring with my hospital clogs.

Finally the phone rang "Hello" I said eagerly. "Hi Dr. Ronco, the cross match is negative, so you can proceed."

I hung up and immediately called Gio's house. "Hi, I'm Claudio from nephrology. Hi Gio'. Here we go — there is a kidney for you. Come to the hospital immediately. Have someone else drive you and here and don't push the Ferrari to two hundred km/hr. It won't be the extra ten minutes that will change your destiny. We are waiting."

Gio' arrived at the hospital and the kidney is already in the operating room. Gio's body is ready to receive the transplant because the dialysis he has just completed at home has served to purify the body. I greeted Gio in the preparation room, while the pre-anesthesia was beginning to take effect. The room smelled of disinfectants and medicines. The lamp projected a cone of light onto the operating field. The green suits of the surgeons made a sharp contrast with the whiteness of the lighting. I let them work and went back to the department where I had other cases to follow. The surgery wound up that morning and they told me that the kidney was already working. The took Gio' to the post-operative ICU and we woke him up calmly. I took a short nap on the cot in the doctor's room and felt as though we had done something good. Gio' and Lara would return to a normal life stronger than ever.

An hour later I woke up to greet my colleague who would be taking over the watch. I told him that I would go home for a shower and would return at the end of the morning to check on the transplant. Stefano, the head of the transplant section would personally follow all the procedures and prescriptions of the first anti-rejection therapies. Gio' was in good hands.

Shortly after noon, I went to the TIPO where my colleagues were waiting for me and shortly began waking him and removing the respirator tube. "Everything is OK," they told me. Gio' opened his eyes and sees me, but still can't speak. He nods his head and blinks his eyes twice that everything was fine and communicated our previously agreed signal that I should go to Lara and tell her that everything was OK. I reached out to her and embraced her as she burst into a liberating cry. The worst was over.

The same evening, I embarked for China leaving Gio' in the hands of our extraordinary team. I hardly even had time to sit on the airplane seat with a pillow under my head and a blanket that led to a restful sleep. I dreamt of Jack Ryan on the hunt for Red October who told the Commander Ranius, as if he were the new Christopher Columbus, "Welcome to your new life, Gio." I murmured in my sound sleep while a stewardess with the delicacy of an angel, added another blanket to me.

Gio' promised that if all went well, he would make a celebration festival — and he did just that. It brought together seven hundred transplant patients and their relatives and friends in an association called "World of Colors" with the aim of forming a group of volunteers to help our ward and those waiting for transplant. Now, we were under a tent in the lawn near the church in his town. The festival had grilled meats and side dishes. A lottery was made to collect proceeds to help cover the expenses. At the end of the party, we managed to raise the necessary funds to pay the salary of a researcher. Gio approached me beaming "you know Doc, at the beginning I had an idea of elegant tables with white tablecloths, candlesticks and a menu of refined foods and champagne. Instead, we find ourselves celebrating with polenta and sausages on wooden planks, but I prefer this a thousand-fold over. I like this because we are more like family as you taught us. All these companions of misfortune — or rather adventure, since they have received the gift of a new life like me, from a great team that will be at your disposal. Just give us a whistle when you need us."

As Gio' left, his mother came to my side "Doctor, I suffered the pains of hell for Giovanni's illness and now I am happy. Only those who pass through it can know what it means.

Giovanni is my life and I will be eternally grateful for what you have done for him."

"Dear Lia," I say "with all the tenderness that I can show you — every patient is my life and Giovanni is also a friend." And since there is not much more to say, we hugged and moved towards the prize stage to see if we have won anything in the lottery. Actually, we are already aware that we have won our "lottery of life" and the prize is Giovanni's transplant.

Gio's transplant had been running for six years and in the meantime, he had Lara had another child. They called him Claudio and I also became his godfather at his baptism. Everything went well until a few months later when Gio's pressure started to go crazy again. This was one of the first signs of a transplanted kidney failure. The prospect now was that possibility of a chronic rejection, for which common therapies are not very effective.

One day Lara came to me with tears in her eyes and asked if there were serious problems. I tried to reassure her, but now she knows me well and I am not able to hide my concern. The picture was complex, and I didn't see a good outcome. I dared not venture into this hypothesis, but if the deterioration of the renal function and uncontrolled pressure continued with the trend, Gio' would soon have serious complications and a high probability to need to return to dialysis. Lara and his mother Lia were desperate.

I proposed a cure with a new drug that seemed to have a moderately positive effect. Gio' came every three days to check and we were able to contain his blood pressure with massive doses of a very powerful drug. We proceed to walk on pins and needles and Gio's equilibrium remained unstable. I tried to also adopt a new therapeutic scheme that had been developed in the US. Gio's condition worsened. His urine became cloudy and progressively reduced in quantity. His skin began to shrivel, and he lost strength and had difficulties breathing. He was anemic and acids in his blood began to rise to dangerous levels.

I suggested that he stay in the hospital for a while so we could better monitor his condition. Gio' was assigned bed 19, in the same room where he had already experienced pains and joy, dramas and rebirth. This time it seemed like the "luck thermometer" was not on his side and trending toward a downward spiral. Every time I passed in front his door, I had less and less desire to enter, because I didn't know what to say. I tried to keep a positive and professional attitude but I also lived this dramatic situation. I had the impression that the kidneys wouldn't work for much longer and that we would have to resume dialysis where we had left off.

The antirejection therapy didn't work.

Gio's kidneys permanently stopped working. In the meantime, my appointment as head of Nephrology and my internship in New York as a professor had given me more confidence in dealing with even the most complicated cases.

I organized a meeting with Stefano, Carlo and Alessandra, my most trusted collaborators and we concluded that the umbilical and inguinal hernias that had appeared on the abdomen precluded the resumption of peritoneal dialysis at home. We would have to set up a vascular access for extracorporeal dialysis. I explained to Gio' and Lara that this was an operation we could perform in our operating room. In reality — it is not such a simple thing, because it is a question of connecting an artery and vein so that the vein becomes turgid and allows an easy puncture with dialysis needles. The intervention is performed on very small vessels of the wrist with threads almost invisible to the bare eye. It is painstaking work that allow us to have access to the blood, circulate and clean it with our filters and then return the clean blood to the patient. This type of dialysis can also be done at home, as long as there is a person who oversees it. Gio' however, doesn't want to involve Lara in this type of activity and agrees to do it in the hospital three times a week. He chooses the afternoon so he can continue to go to the factory in the morning.

Gio's condition worsened and after only a few days since the fistula surgery on the left wrist, it was necessary for him to start extracorporeal dialysis. Fortunately, he tolerated the treatment well and no imbalances were observed. Fifteen days later Gio was in much better shape. Even though he currently had three kidneys, not even one was working. Thus, he began a new period of his life with the rhythms marked by the dialysis session three times a week. "Claudio" he told me one day "how is that miniaturization project for the artificial kidney to make it portable and wearable going?" "Do you think I would be able to try it?." I told him that we were still the beginning and working on a prototype in the laboratory and that we were still not able to test it in humans.

"How long will it take?" he asked me.

"Dear Gio," I replied, it is not just a matter of time, but more of funding, and as you know, our country is not generous with research funding. We can do everything possible, but I am not able to make predictions. We are collaborating with a group in the Netherlands and one in the US, and we also have a good collaboration with the Mechanical Engineering Institute in Vicenza. We will put in double the effort to see if you might become the first patient."

One year later we were ready to try the first experiment for the wearable artificial kidney. I called Gio' by phone and invited him to the hospital. "We will do a test on six patients including you, but don't get too excited, as there are many years from the first experiments to being ready for routine applications.

Gio' replied "It doesn't matter. I will arrive as soon as possible. Can't wait to try this device of yours."

The experiment was deemed a success and Gio' was the first patient in the world to walk wearing a functioning artificial kidney. Battery life required us to stop after eight hours, but it was definitely on the right track. The data was shared around the world and Gio' was satisfied to have contributed to this step forward in an attempt to free patients from the slavery of being tied to a machine three times a week for the dialysis session.

I pointed out to Gio', in this moment of enthusiasm, that now he had to go back to reality of his usual dialysis regime, hoping for a new transplant.

Gio' had undergone an ultrasound to check on the general condition of the vessels and abdomen in view of a second transplant. We observed a mass that didn't appear to be a cyst and we needed to investigate this. "Gio'," I told him, "we need to do a CT scan with contrast medium and perhaps also a MRI. Do you understand what we are talking about? We need to get to the bottom of this."

He looked at me apprehensively. Everything always seemed to happen to him. I thought he might be on the verge of a nervous breakdown and despair, but then stood up proudly and declared "Come on Doc, let's face this too. Stay close and you will see it will be all right.

I was almost frightened by his ability to accept the misfortunes that fate always reserved for him, but it seemed like he knew how to transform these into challenges. CT and resonance confirmed the diagnostic suspicion. He had a tumor that was small, but certainly malignant, that needed to be removed. I explained this to Lara and his mother Lia and told them that the operation will not fortunately be complex and since we are already here, it could also be considered as an opportunity to do something useful for a future transplant.

We went into the room together and I said to Gio' "We need to take away one of your old kidneys, which in any case aren't useful since they no longer function, and at the same time we will also take away the kidney you had received as a gift from the transplant in order to make room for a new kidney for a future transplant." I didn't have the courage to give the full details. The presence of a tumor such as the one that Gio' had, usually require an observation period of three years in which it isn't possible to be considered for a transplant. In fact, if the tumor is fully removed, the immunosuppressive drugs that are administered after the transplant could facilitate a relapse. Our immune system, in addition to keeping bacteria, viruses and many other things in check, also kills thousands of cancer cells every day — which avoids that they proliferate. When we give drugs to increase the tolerance to the transplanted kidney to limit rejection, we also simultaneously decrease our natural defenses. This is why Giovanni with his new pathology, would need to be excluded from the transplant list for at least three years, as the best-case scenario if all went well.

Bad luck had really plagued poor Gio'.

***

Three long years had passed, and Gio' had been forced into a life regimen full of cautions to avoid compromising the results of dialysis. It is analogous to driving a boat in dry conditions and navigating between the salt marshes, the canals and the shallows of the Venetian lagoons.

One day I called Gio' on the phone and asked him to come to the hospital for an extra check-up. He arrived, accompanied by Lara. These days he was a little bent and walked with his feet dragging a bit. He seemed to have a weight on his shoulders from the years of dialysis and long series of disappointments and misadventures. The exams are good however and his health is discrete with a good correction of renal failure.

"Gio," I tell him, "we are out of the shallows! Three years have passed since that damned unexpected event and the last CT is perfect. You seem completely cured and there are no other signs of the tumor. I can put you back on the list for transplantation. But before you tell me anything, I must inform you that this time, the kidney will not come to you from a stranger and unwitting donor. It will come to you from a person who gave you life the first time. Lia, your mother, has already done all the compatibility tests and exams and has proved to be a perfect donor for you. There are no other obstacles. Despite her slightly advanced age, she is in great health and her kidneys are in excellent shape. We will do a living donor transplant, and mamma Lia will give you one of her kidneys."

Gio' broke down in uncontrollable tears.

"We kept this from you, because until the last minute, we weren't sure how things would go. Both Lara and Lia offered to be donors, but Lara turned out to be an incompatible donor, while Lia presented "four compatibilities." You will need to do two more months of dialysis, then we will proceed with the surgery. The previous operation has fixed your abdomen, so you should be able to receive the new kidney without any problems."

"Doc, I don't know, I don't know if I can accept this gift from my mother. She has done too much for me. It isn't right."

"Dear Gio', I will take care of the clinical part and the rest you will need to discuss between yourselves. Knowing your mom — It doesn't seem likely that she will change her mind, so it is best to talk to her and best wishes. Remember though, that the gift you receive from her will be nothing in comparison to the gift you will give her in making her happy about your new life."

At the end, Lia quickly put an end to Gio's resistance by stating a stern, "Do as I say and that is it. Enough!"

On the 4th of April, almost four years and a few months from when Gio' had started dialysis we were finally ready. The compatibility showed promise that the transplant would succeed and have a high probability for long term success. Lia had no underlying pathologies and we checked her head to foot. She had an appendicitis as a young woman — but nothing else. She was as healthy as you could be, and it was apparent to all that she was pushing this forward with love and determination. All third parties that were consulted ascertained that her desire to donate was appropriate and motivated out of true love and approved the possibility for donation.

Gio' was on the stretcher in front of the operating room with his mother beside him. They were like poetry to behold. It seemed like not too much time had passed that they once in a delivery room and now together in the operating room. Pre-sedation procedures began shortly before the actual anesthesia. I looked in and saw the look of love and determination in Lia's eyes; and I saw in Gio' his great hope and gratitude for the woman who is about to give his life again a second chance.

"Gio," I say, "If all goes well, we will have a great party."

"If all goes well Doc, I think we should have a party ten times the one we had the first time and invite all the transplant patients who are part of our large family. Stay here and don't leave me alone, Doc. I'd like to wake up with the good news that I am peeing again, and you have to be here to give this news to me. I don't trust anyone else."

The operation began, but right away it was noted that there were some unexpected complexities due to some anomalies in the vasculature. The surgeon was an expert however and overcame the obstacles. Lia's kidney was in perfect condition. Once implanted into Gio's body, it began to work immediately. In transplants from a corpse donor, there is always the unknown factor of some small damage suffered by the kidney for the time elapsed since removing the organ and implantation. This isn't a problem in living donors because everything is programmed like a stopwatch. After a few hours, Gio' is transferred to postoperative intensive care. I tiptoed into the room full of monitors and equipment and found the ICU chief who told me he wanted to scale down the sedation and slowly wake up the patient.

These were moments that were always difficult to predict,

nor become accustomed. Shortly before, I had gone to find Lia who had already been awake and had targeted me with a barrage of questions about her son's transplant. I calmed the courageous mother down and now could dedicate myself completely to Gio' — patient, friend and member of our large family. There was a cough when the tube was extracted from his airway with labored breathing. His chest struggled as it was no longer helped by the mechanical respirator. There was also a period of a state of consciousness that comes and goes with a corresponding response of the heart rhythm to the new stimuli that are perceived after the withdrawal from the anesthesia.

Gio's eyes opened to scan the surrounding world — a new world made of new sensations and emotions. I shook his hand. Gio' still couldn't speak and he questioned me with his eyes. I told him softly, "Your mom is fine, and you are making a lot of urine. The operation went well and there couldn't have been a better kidney in the world than the one you received from "mamma Lia."

There were no words to describe that moment — but it firmly entrenches and whispers to your unconscious being the thousand reasons why being a doctor is something unique. Not that there is a need for this, because for each fall, a doctor will find the strength to get up and at each failure a new life returns to give hope and pushes for the cycle to never stop. In some fleeting moments, you have the perception to change the trajectory from a life descending a steep slope from despair towards joy.

"Doc, I remind you of my big celebration. You cannot miss it even if the Pope in person would come to visit you that day."

For me, and unaware to Gio', I have already celebrated, with the first drop of urine with the new kidney.

Cooking healthy for the kidneys

SUNDAY EVENINGS my father always decided the menu for the week. We had boiled meat on Wednesdays, meatballs on Thursdays and Bacala' on Fridays. Lunches and dinners were organized on the basis of what had been given to the doctor — particularly eggs and poultry, so that nothing was wasted. Il Toni of the contrada busa district sent us tagliatelle that his wife had prepared, Giuseppe the cheesemaker sent us cheese and Bruno would send us game hen. These were from his courtyard and were so tough that, to be able to eat them, you would need to dry age and plan their cooking well in advance. While I took the skills of organizing the moments of the dinner from my father, I learned the culinary techniques from my mother. At that time of my life in Asiago, slow cooking at low temperatures, which is so fashionable today, was done daily thanks to our old stove. The range had a large cast-iron center plate that was always hot and allowed us to cook at different temperatures, depending on necessity. We could cook with a lively heat for polenta or with a slow constant heat for bacala'. It was enough to just find the right spot on the cast-iron plate.

Over the years I have always nourished my passion for gastronomy by exploring traditional as well as modern gastronomic recipes. I've met chefs, hosts and innkeepers, acclaimed restaurateurs and wine experts. I've learned something from everyone. Afterall, what could be better than returning from a long night of shift work and passing by the butcher shop to buy a priest's hat for a pot roast or a round steak for veal with tuna sauce?

What can be better to help me forget, at least for a moment, the diseases and suffering that follow me home, as when oil is distributed in the pan and the onion begins to take on a slow translucent hue with pieces of meat browned with high heat and then slowly cooked together with wine and vegetables. Or more relaxing than preparing onion with anchovies spread over pieces of cod in a terracotta container with milk and a little cheese and then slowly simmering this according to the official recipe as suggested by the Venerable Brotherhood of Bacala' alla Vicentina? But if these breaks in the kitchen are so useful to me to catch my breath and regenerate the days complicated by the psychological burden of the suffering of others that becomes unbearable when you lose a patient who had become your friend, why not also try to think of something that might also raise the morale of patients?

Although I have followed the problems of renal patients and their diseases for many years, at the forefront, I have tried to think of patients as individuals with their own world, their own reality and specific problems to be solved. In my long experience, I have learned a lot by listening to stories of patients and their families, so much so that today I consider the collection of clinical anamneses perhaps the most important moment of the diagnosis and treatment. Sometimes symptoms and syndromes are better described by the patients themselves than by the manuals of even highly qualified authors.

Sometimes, apparently insignificant ailments or abnormalities turn out to be unmistakable signs of a problem thanks to the courage of patients speaking up and sharing in-depth details with a trusted doctor. This is particularly true for kidney diseases which are often insidious and can lead to severe organ failure without the person noticing or manifesting obvious symptoms. Even in cases of timely and precise diagnoses, element of doubt or suspicion about something wrong with the treatment can be picked up by the doctor during a conversation with a patient, perhaps after he has taken off the white coat and hung it on the coat rack.

Among the aspects we know today as complex intricate nature of chronic kidney disease, diet and nutrition undoubtably represent one of the aspects that are most easily overlooked. Small eating disorders, allergies, intolerances, refusal of some foods, inability to swallow, dry mouth, nausea and postprandial weight on the stomach are often overlooked or underestimated. The cause may lie either in the superficial manner of collecting the patient information, or in the unconscious underestimation of the phenomenon by the patient himself who tends not to fully disclose the problem and often dismisses its severity.

Chronic kidney disease goes through several stages during which the intake of nutrients and the prescribed diet can vary significantly. The picture is further complicated if there are concomitant comorbidities such as diabetes, gout, or other metabolic dysfunctions. As a result, the nephropathic patient often renounces feeding properly for fear of ingesting harmful substances, or worse still, not eating at all due to lack of knowing which foods are allowed, recommended or compatible. There is quite a bit of information on the diet for dialysis patients, but the writings that directly address them and their families often lack advice on how to shop, how to cook food and how to prepare the most appropriate dishes. Above all, there are no books that suggest how to make lunch or dinner a joyful moment, despite the inevitable vetoes and deprivations imposed on their diets to keep the levels of phosphorous, potassium, etc. under control.

One of the biggest difficulties for nephropathic patients is the constant sensation of thirst, which is partly a real physical phenomena and partly psychological due to the restrictions on liquid intake for fear of having too much weight gain between dialysis sessions with the consequence of longer sessions to dispose of the excess weight. All this means that the patient often prefers a hundred grams of water rather than the same amount in carbohydrates, fats and proteins, sometimes leading to a serious state of malnutrition.

For this reason, I decided to do something also for the dialysis "kitchen." The opportunity presented itself to me last autumn when together with a group of volunteers from our association, I thought about the Christmas gifts to be given to our hospitalized patients, to make them feel part of our large family.

For many years, as a delegate of the Italian Academy of Cuisine of Vicenza, I have been committed to keeping the food and wine culture of our territory alive, by rediscovering food, recipes and ancient traditions. I am an avid supporter of the value of a "shared table" and I sustain the belief that food and meals not shared cause a great loss in the value of the food itself. The ancient Romans said, "It doesn't matter what you eat, but who you eat with." If this is true for the healthy population, then imagine how a patient feels when seated at a table and forced to face a diet full of prohibitions and deprivations. Why should they renounce the modest pleasures of a "shared table." Is it really true that kidney disease is incompatible with the passion for pots and pans? My idea was further born from meetings and support from extraordinary people such as Marco the pharmacist, Natascia the dietician, Vanessa — our student doing a thesis in the field of nutrition, the young nephrologist — Laura and Claudia, an expert in food preparation. The idea was to make a simple unpretentious book that could help nephropathic patients and their families feel "less different" in the kitchen and at the table, especially for special occasions such as Christmas. We involved the help of a true culinary star of food and wine, Alfredo Pelle, president of the Study Center of the Italian Academy of Cuisine (Accademia Italiana della Cucina), a great man and friend, and last but not least, also one of our dialysis patients.

Aflredo shared with us the sentiments and problems that dialysis patients face and showed us that the kitchen for dialysis patients can range from home stoves to sophisticated equipment used by professionals in the sector. In fact, he asked some star chefs to contribute to the volume with the author's recipes compatible with nephrologic diseases. He also asked Arrigo Cipriani, an extraordinary and ingenious man, that embodied quality of raw materials and simplicity for recipes, to write the introduction. The book *"La buona cucina per I reni"*(Healthy Cooking for the Kidneys) came out in 2018 (Padova, Piccin) and was dedicated as follows:

> *I dedicate this to you, my patient and friend. Don't feel sad about the rigid dietary restrictions, but rather focus on the creative joys of eating in the company of loved ones at the home dinner table. You don't have to give up the desire for a normal life if you want to fight kidney disease. To face the treatment with dialysis in the best way and obtain the maximum benefit, you must take care of nutrition, which is a real medicine for you. Nutrition is important for maintaining muscle mass, red blood cells and the immune system. You must feed yourself and feed yourself well. You will be able to do it if you use intelligence and sometimes creativity, avoiding some foods and favoring others. Fortunately, Italy is full of food varieties that allow a personalized zero-kilometer gastronomy. This is what you have to look for in the maze of dietary recommendations and restrictions. This book will help you to discover recipes that will seem unthinkable or even obsolete, but that will allow you to invent a creative gastronomy full of flavors and emotions. From our book, you can learn how to make and enjoy incredible recipes without even disturbing your metabolic balance and cure that your condition requires. I*

hope that this book will allow you to reconsider the joy of cooking and celebration of food that you may have lost or thought you might have to abandon. The objective of this book is to add a place at the table for those that suffer from renal disease, without feeling different from others. That person is you. We want you to be included as our friends and diners, and not just patients.

IV. From the past to the future

"Buon maestro è chi avrà generato un allievo
in grado di superarlo."

A good teacher is one that generates students
able to overcome him.

—*Giovanni A. Barraco*

Teachers and mentors

A MENTOR IS a constant beacon present at various moments in the student's life. Enthusiasm and choices depend on the mentor to overcome and the ability to help overcome difficulties. The mentor is not a professor, but rather a life teacher.

My first real teacher was Giuseppe La Greca, head of the nephrology department at the Vicenza Hospital when I entered in 1976 as a substitute. La Greca was a brilliant, intelligent and wise man who radiated great charisma. He had become chief of the department when he was just 34 years old from Parma. The president of the Vicenza hospital, Dr. Fanton, had gone to choose him from one of the group of students from Professor Migone, whose studies were known worldwide. La Greca, from Southern Italy, had integrated into the difficult and closed Vicenza community thanks to his expansive relationship skills and good-naturedness. He taught me everything he knew about nephrology, and above all, in the times when the "old guard" prevented young collaborators from being protagonists in their specialist discipline. He gave me ample research space by stimulating me enough and at the same time, holding me back if I was too hasty. These were daily life lessons that I can't forget.

Towards the end of his career, our relationship broke down because La Greca had not accepted the idea that I would replace him once he retired, even though, he himself had promoted me to the competition. He saw me as his successor and at the same as the one who would be "stealing" his place. It was an irrational feeling and therefore understandable and excusable.

In any case, I am very grateful to him and hope I have honored his work as a master by continuing to grow the department that he created in the way that also seemed better to me. I have already mentioned my second mentor, Juan Bosch. He was the person that welcomed me during my first stay in the US. He was from Chile and had attended medical school in Santiago, and then went to the US. How could I describe Juan? Genius and unruliness, distraction and intuition, brilliant disorder and methodical lack of attention to detail, but also the person that profoundly changed my life. He taught me to do research and not just fall in love with my ideas when other showed me that they were wrong. He pushed me towards scientific methodology without letting me lose sight of the values of humanism. With him, I understood that you have to be simple in communicating and not worry about showing everything you know. Juan taught me the difference between a good and a great doctor.

"Claudio," he told me "remember that the one who is not generous, is not great. Don't be afraid to communicate your intuitions and ideas to others. Maybe the idea will become developed or even better, even if that person was not even the one that had the original idea. Tomorrow you will have another and then another still. Don't keep distance between your colleagues and students. Let them become as close as possible. The smart few who reach you, may even exceed your strengths and become your pride and joy. The others will be harmless and useless."

The third teacher that changed my life was Nathan Levin, who in two years transformed me from a mere doctor-researcher to a doctor-professor and mentor. Nathan had pushed me to realize that I could be a central point for fellows, in much the same way that Juan had been for me several years before. He gave me full freedom to manage all of the operations of the Institute. When I decided to leave the United Stated and return to Vicenza, he gave me his heartfelt wishes; "Claudio, you have a grand gift to stimulate all to work together — to row in the same direction and with the same rhythm (he had been on the Cambridge rowing team). I'm sorry you will leave us, but your destiny seems set on a course. You will always be looking for someone to train and someone to convey your enthusiasm and desire to get things done."

***

My colleagues from the University of California San Diego (UCSD), presented me with a career award and introduced me as a pioneer of new dialysis techniques for critically ill patients. I jokingly replied as I started my lecture, that when they define you as a pioneer, they are only secretly declaring that you are old, because the term itself has the concept of discoveries and research conducted over a long period of time. To be defined as a pioneer of something in the future, you must have the courage today — or have had it yesterday - to follow your intuitions and thoughts as perceived as too innovative. I told them that in my personal case, in 1990 I had sent one of my publications to a scientific journal that rejected it without appeal. They judged my theory of application of new imaging techniques to newly conceived medical devices as "not interesting." Ten years later, I rediscovered that work and sent it back to the same journal. What do you know? They accepted it with lots of compliments for the novelty of my conclusions. If they had published it then, today I would be the pioneer of the theory I presented.

What characterizes the true pioneer are intuition and

strength of coherence, without of course, going beyond stubbornness, the discrimination of stupidity. But there is also no doubt that to become a pioneer in a scientific discipline also takes luck. Being in the right place at the right time. This was also my case. I had arrived in New York when my colleagues were starting an experiment on new dialysis membranes. I had been assigned to a different project, but since I realized that membrane research had a greater development potential, I offered to follow this. Now, thirty years later after discussing the clinical applications of those membranes, I have turned out to be the greatest expert and in a certain sense the father of the new perspectives.

The pioneers of a discipline, even if they are not our tutors, should represent an important focal point for us scholars. We must consider them "distant masters." I had the honor and pleasure of meeting several pioneers of my discipline," Pim Kolff, the inventor of the artificial kidney; Belding Scribner, the father of modern dialysis — both who are exemplary models of simplicity and modesty; Eric Drexler, the father of nanotechnology who was crazy like a horse. These men had an enormous influence and my success was in part because of opportunities afforded by these encounters. I tried to adsorb every drop of their knowledge to discover the secret of their intuitions and imagine their paths. In addition, from these and from other great scientists, I learned the ability to recognize not only the positive things that were done, but also the usefulness of mistakes over time. None of them were ashamed of their mistakes and indeed they often considered mistakes as useful and sometimes as indispensable for their discoveries. Without this valuable lesson, I would not have in turn become a tutor worthy of the name, with the possibility to become an example and stimulus for students and increase their self-esteem in the face of the inevitable ways that the game plays out, also with mistakes.

Irrivians forever!

"HI LADIES, how are things going?" I say entering the laboratory. "What is the latest news regarding the thesis?

"We are at a good point" replies Anna, while Martina, always shy and reserved remains silent. Anna is a bioengineer who has been working with me for almost five years. She asked me for an interview after a TED talk in Padova because, - she told me - she was fascinated by my way of telling the recent progress of nephrology. She wanted to join our group and be able to actively participate, she hoped, as a protagonist, in scientific progress. Anna is the tutor of Martina, a bioengineering student sent to me for an experimental thesis by my colleague from Padova, teacher of the biomaterials course. Together we had carried out research on a new dialysis membrane that should have better characteristics than those used so far. In the last five months, we have been side -by-side performing experiments, trying solutions and testing new materials amid disappointments, bitterness, enthusiasm, and some success. Our meetings and discussions were done mainly in the evenings, since during the day I was completely busy with the routine clinical work.

"I brought some dessert pastries that they gave to me in Iran" I said smiling. I just got back from a long and tiring flight, but this evening with you helped me forget about all that. The pastries are made up of honey almonds and pistachios. Rich in calories, just to refuel your brains from which I smell the emission of a burnt odor."

My joke softened the air. I want them to be completely relaxed before tackling the problems of my student's thesis. I begin to tell them about the thesis, that I did in Padua many years ago. "It seemed an extraordinary thing to do an experimental thesis like you are doing, dear Martina. I realized that it was an absolute novelty for the Faculty of Medicine. It would have been original, new, perhaps even good. The same enthusiasm and emotion I felt a few years later with the specialty thesis. I was already in the hospital, and doing a little research and continuing to study. It seemed like a dream. I had to leave the academy for survival. My father had fallen ill, and there was no money to run the family. I accepted the job that had been offered to me. My professor accused me of having betrayed the scientific cause and of selling myself to hospital medicine, but I continued to study as though I had stayed inside the university walls — just as I have continued to do today."

"Is that why you spend your evenings with us and care about us so much?" Martina asked me with a surge of enthusiasm.

"You see Martina, research and studies are like a hockey game. You can watch it from the grandstand and wait for the result, or you can play it yourself. But no matter what the role, if you decide to play you have to put your heart into it and play it all the way. And when you feel you are ready, not only to play, but also teach, then you can be a coach. The transition from player to coach is as difficult as the transition between doing and getting things done. At the beginning, it seems that nobody can do things as well as you do, but as time goes on, you learn to delegate and find that even the student in the back row has a will to do things, with hidden energy and an overflowing imagination. And if at that moment, you decide to entrust him with a task that will absolutely floor you with novelty and creativity. And this is how science and research evolve. The youngest take the baton from the teacher, as in a relay race. In turn they become masters of science and life."

We then come back down to earth to face the problems of Martina's thesis. Anna tells me about the instability of the biochemical tests. Martina tells me that the statistics are a bit weak. The discussion should be reviewed based on the results obtained and the potential for new future research.

As I look at my two young students, the *Gaudeamus igitur* (let us rejoice) of De brevitate vitae, the international song of the university study, whirls in my head. I can hear the choruses that are coming: Vivat Academia, vivant Professores!"

With that music in mind, I say goodbye to the girls and leave them to their calculations. After all, they are always engineers and a little mathematics is needed in our world of cells, molecules and human emotions. Between a test, research and thesis work, I can stay close to my students, and continue to be, in my own way, a perpetual student.

More than a hundred young people have come to Vicenza from all over the world to do research in our **IRRIV** *(International Renal Research Institute Vicenza)*. Clean faces, innocent eyes and strong will. Whether they come from China, America, Israel, Mexico, Thailand or Norway, they all share the same passion for study and innovation.

We meet every Monday for a group meeting. Everyone brings ideas, projects, new developments or newly published scientific articles. We are like the group of young people at the mountain districts who play and grow in the courtyard between the houses. Over the years, pastimes and players change and the group is renewed. When someone grows up and becomes too old to stay with the others, he goes out and another comes in to take that place. Our scientific community is much the same, it is renewed every year. We average about ten people in our meetings and almost every month have a party for those who will return to their country or for the new ones who join the group. In this way, our community expands dramatically, because those who return home stay in touch. We become researchers of a global village based all over the world.

One morning we were sitting around the meeting room table and I listened to the various problems and challenges they were encountering. Mauro talked to me about his difficulties in terms of mathematical models. Anna has encountered problems for the software of the new equipment. The reagents for Erik's study are too expensive, the study proposed by Ignacio could take ten years before the ethics committee approval, the analyses for the kidney damage biomarker proposed by Ghada are taking too long — but need to go on. Others inform me that the flow cytometer has broken, that the funds for the cardiovascular monitor are still blocked, that Faeq's multicenter study requires further analysis before he leaves and that the devices for the new extracorporeal therapies must pass the biocompatibility test.

I see that in the face of these difficulties, the group is a bit downcast. They need a healthy boost. Then I look them in the eye and in our "Euro English" which is the common language of the scientific world, I say to them "Guys, it is true we lack resources and sometimes hindered by bureaucracy, but we must stay strong. We can't give up. If some projects go slowly, we can have others that proceed in parallel. If one stops, we will replace it with another. We will circumvent the blocks by activating alternative ways as we do in the network. We don't lack ideas. You see, research is basically like a game. Toys are not enough to play. It takes creativity, curiosity, intuition, initiative and, above all, will. If you were to ask me if it was possible to someday win the Nobel prize, I would reply that it would be difficult, but not impossible. Why set limits for ourselves? We imagine, work, study, invent solutions. Our catchphrase is "innovention and innovaction," that is, we invent innovation and put a maximum effort to achieve this. Our research is a game and it must keep us amused. For each problem, we imagine an experiment with multiple solutions. Tony will focus on solution A, Asuman on B. And when we run out of resources, let's not think too much about that and make sure we don't lose our spirit. Research is an important game and whoever wins improves the lives of patients. Let's keep playing. As my hockey teammates say "the only goal you will never score is what you haven't tried to do. If you don't shoot you don't score. So, build the action, go from defense to attack. Pass information as players pass the puck. Get close to the door and "slap" a nice shot. Some discs will end up outside, some will be blocked by the goalkeeper of bureaucracy or misery, but some will end up in the net and you will have scored the goal. Many of our fellows today are professors at their Universities because they did not give up and continued to play the game, even when it seemed lost."

These fellows of mine, away from home and with meager stipends, would have every reason to be depressed, but they know they are playing in a courageous, imaginative and unprejudiced team, and the coach's blow made them understand that they will not be able to breathe until they will have made the goal of their life. *"Made our oars wings,"* would have been how this would have been concluded by Dante.

Our fellows have literally colonized the world. At the entrance to the Singapore General Hospital, there is a plaque that declares: "This department was created after the Vicenza Model." At the Jiao Tong University of Shanghai, my former fellow Lu made a replica of our model of the IRRIV and the meeting room is practically identical to ours. In Greece, the director, Dimitri, of Cardio nephrology of the Onassis cardiac surgery center, was a fellow and Emilio is the director of the Nephrology department of Ioannina. In Thailand, in Bangkok, Ranitta is a professor of nephrology at the University, while Dusit in Chiang Mai manages the critical nephrology center. At the cardiology institute of Mexico, where modern cardiolgy was born, Armando is becoming the contact person for the cardiorenal syndrome that we discovered and defined in Vincenza. In San Diego Dinna Cruz became a staff member of the University of Southern California in San Diego after spending seven years with us in Vicenza and having published some of the most interesting research in our sector. I meet my former students and fellows in every corner of the world. Helsinki, Giessen, Hyderabad, Moscow, Melbourne, Pittsburgh. These are all locations where I periodically meet my (scientific) children. They are affectionate and welcome me like the pope. In Rome, they compete to organize "cacio e pepe"; in Beijing, they spoil me with Peking duck, the best sushi is reserved for me in Tokyo and I am sure to have the classic 2 finger high steak when in Pittsburgh. My fellows are my satisfaction and success. Through them, I have crossed borders and oceans. I reached remote continents sharing knowledge and ways of thinking. I can't say if I enriched them, or they enriched me. But one thing they all repeat in their social networks: that Vicenza was not just a school of nephrology for them. It was a school of life. Everyone feels they have something in common. Everyone calls themselves Irrivians, that is, students of **IRRIV**. And as you know, *Irrivians are forever.*

If you've been an Irrivian, you will be forever.

Gaudeamus igitur

AT THE UNIVERSITY, what I really missed, was having a good master teacher. I had good instructors such as Professor Austoni, a renowned semiologist; Professor Fiaschi — a passionate, but gruff teacher, Professor Zatti, a genius capable of making us love physiology, the human body and functions. While you could say that these were good teachers, and probably could have been even great teachers, if it hadn't been for the large workload and high number of students attending their courses not preventing them from having a direct and personal relationship with us students. Nonetheless, I continue to have an unconditional passion for the University. I have always loved the environment and the spirit of academics. I have always liked students and student spirit anywhere in the world.

I fondly remember my various trips to foreign Universities. Valladolid, where the large colonnade in front of the main office has represented an insurmountable limit for the police for centuries; at the University of Virginia with the sprawling green lawn on the Charlottesville campus surrounded by the portico of the student dorm rooms and offices of professors. One of my great dreams during my retirement is to travel around the world to visit Universities found on the four corners of the planet. I want to see their libraries, rectorate rooms and to understand how others understand the Academy. I want to meet the deans, see the founding documents and understand the sporting traditions, the songs and the illustrious personalities shown in the cases and displays all within the walls of the illustrious halls of such prestigious institutions such as Oxford, Cambridge, Montpellier and Valladolid.

I always dreamed of being able to teach at the University and to be among students. I wanted to understand their uncertainties, their curiosities and to help them grow. Improve and study with them to advance on the path of science without losing the zest for life and rejoice in youth as Patty Pravo sang the "world that will host us" in Sad Boy. I have always suffered from not being able to carry out a mission for which I seem to be suited and that I consider to be among the most noble and useful. Students keep you alive and young. The academy is not an abstract thing, it is a way of living and making your students live. It is a way of leaving some of you in the world to come. This is why I created IRRIV, and for this, I fought to get our department recognized as an official clinical part of the University. IRRIV is now an official part of the University of Padova and will survive after I retire. The dream cultivated for many long years, and to return within the walls of the University of Padua where I studied, and where the great giants of science, not the least Galileo taught, had finally come true. I have finally entered the ranks of the teaching staff of the University of Padua as a full professor. All these years to study, publish, specialize. Finally the University called me with the maximum title: Full professor with distinguished honor. I never would have thought that I could have finally arrived at this point. I had received honors, honorary degrees, external roles in Shanghai and Beijing. Even a full professorship in the United

States, but I never thought I could finally realize my dream of becoming a Full Professor at my University.

It was done, and we had arrived at the day of the exam. But this time, it wasn't like all the other numerous exams I had done in my life: second and fifth grade, in the fifth gymnasium, in the third year of high school and then with the exams of the specialization courses for medicine and professional entrance exams. This was my first exam as a teacher.

The nine registered students were waiting for me in the Nievo room on the ground floor after the Ancient Courtyard of the Palazzo Bo, the heart of our University. Before the building became the central structure of the University in 1222, the year of its foundation, it had housed an inn, shops and what was called *Hospitium Bovis* — perhaps an area used to house cattle. It was only in the sixteenth century that it took on its present form with the Ancient Courtyard highlighted by a double row of columns that are always fascinating to observe. The walls of the portico are literally covered with the coats of arms of the families of academics and ancient students, who funded the professor salaries, thus ensuring their full freedom from religious or political interferences. Padua in fact, was the first "University of students," with a secular approach to knowledge that was unprecedented.

Since I had arrived early, I took the time to go upstairs to see the Coats of Arms and epitaphs that were also along the main staircase and in the loggia overlooking from above. An inscription recalls Elena Lucrezia Cornaro Piscopia, a Venetian nobleman, the first woman in the world to graduate. It was 1678 and she graduated in Philosophy, since the discussion of the thesis was precluded in her specialty, theology, which was not admissible then for a woman. How times have changed! Today, many more women than men graduate in Medicine and the profession of "doctor" is returning to the hands of the fairer sex, as it was in the ancient world, when Egyptian pharaohs, Athenian oligarchs and roman emperors preferred to put their health in the hands of female doctors and surgeons.

The classroom door located in the west wing of the porch is open. Within a moment, the busts and frescoes, some of them even disturbing appear. In that room, I too was declared a Doctor of Medicine, "for the powers conferred on me by the Magnificent Rector." To not give in to nostalgia, I hurry to go along another corridor that leads to the Great Hall where the inauguration of the Academic Year has been celebrated for centuries. It is imposing and austere, full of suggestions. Already in 1939, as a classroom reserved for jurists, it was exceptionally granted to Galileo Galilei for the influx of students to his lessons. A chair from the lectures is still preserved today in the nearby Sala Dei Quaranta. Immediately afterwards I found myself admiring the famous anatomical theater designed for the practical lessons of pathologic anatomy by Girolamo Fabrici d'Acquapendente. It has a dizzying wooden architecture in the shape of an inverted cone with different orders of balconies that allowed all present to view the anatomical pieces sectioned by the professor.

I try and imagine what the courses of those illustrious colleagues of mine could have been. Certainly unique, if students from all over Europe came to attend them, as evidenced by the coats of arms of the Ancient Courtyard and the Great Hall. Influenced by them, Masters of science and teaching, I tried to draw my own inspiration and to organize my first course, trying to keep in mind that a professor is there for the students and not vice versa. Just like the first days of the University of Padua, students could still reject professors that they felt were not up to par. To excite the curiosity and increase the attention of my modern students, I resorted to all the resources a researcher and mentor that I had available in my hospital experience and IRRIV. I often highlighted the lessons with anecdotes of life and information that couldn't be found in books. I keep their interest awake with demonstrations of live interventions, or didactic simulations where we illustrate cases and give them the role of a specialist (radiologist, cardiologist, nephrologist, laboratory physician or internist). I also instilled in them the need to know how to speak to specialists from non-medical disciplines. In short, I tried to go beyond the kidney specialist and to make my lessons a *school of life*.

I returned to the ground floor and entered the exam room. The nine candidates are a little agitated, so I try and help them by setting up the test as if it were a chat between colleagues, a discussion at the patient's bed and almost a collective summary of the subject. An easy way of dealing with problems by sharing knowledge. Sharing ignorance and multiplying knowledge has always been my motto. The marks are excellent, with some thirty (highest score) and thirty with honors. I take this opportunity for one last warning: "Guys — I say, thirty in nephrology has little meaning if considered by itself. On the other hand, it is important if you consider it a commitment to maintain over time, and for each future patient, that quality of knowledge and study that has led you to today's excellent result." Contrary to the clichés that circulate about young people, I believe that our current students are extraordinary in commitment and maturity and better than we were. They have a more difficult task than ours — that of coping with a more difficult society and an extremely more complex profession. I am convinced that the future will be in good hands with them. I am happy and confident, and I invite them to celebrate with a spritz at the Pedrocchi café. I find myself humming the words of the *Gaudeamus igitur*: "pereat tristitia pereant osores!" Down with sadness and those that don't have goodness at heart.

V. Live life to the fullest

"There is no passion to be found playing small — in settling for a life that is less than the one you are capable of living." (You can't find passion by living in a mediocre manner)

—*Nelson Mandela*

Notes from the heart

WE MAKE A BIG effort at the IRRIV to publicize how dramatic kidney disease can be and the importance of research. We need many resources to ensure our research and provide scholarships for Irrivians. We have done this by involving different charities and categories of associations: Lions, Carabinieri (police) and even the Lanerossi Vicenza football team. The two major events that organize successfully every year are the rock concert with the Checco Corona band and the hockey game with the legendary Asiago. There are stories that personally concern me and go so far back in time, that the reader may not even want to know.

The person who knows how to read music, can read the language of angels. I was always fascinated by the dense scores, staffs, black dots, keys, expressions and signs from which musicians bring out incredible melodies with their instruments. But even more, I was fascinated by the composers who lowered their emotions and ideas in those notes.

It was the evening of Holy Saturday in 1957 and just like every year, we attended the Easter vigil. I was with my uncle Gigi at nine o'clock in the evening and went to follow him to the San Matteo Cathedral of Asiago. We were continually getting up and kneeling during the Passion according to the Levate and flectamus genua pronounced by the celebrant.

But I lived in anticipation of the singing of the *Gloria*. The *Gloria in Excelsis Deo* underlines the most important moment of the liturgical year, the moment of Christ's resurrection and redemption of Christians.

The *Gloria* was excluded from the masses of Lent, which was noted as a period of sadness and pain. It reappeared in the solemn Easter mass with all its disruptive joy around ten o'clock. At that moment, the purple drapes that had obscured sacred statues and paintings during Lent fell. The bells, which also remained silent for forty days, were loosened and rang triumphantly mixing with the Argentine din of all the bells of various timbres and shades shaken madly by the altar boys, while the faithful at home, according to tradition, bathed eyes to remember Mary's tears. The solemn mass was accompanied by the pipe organ, one of the largest in the Vicenza province.

That evening my uncle Gigi had brought me behind the altar so I could see the organist Tullio who, having adjusted the registers on the "strong" and "very strong," pounded on the keys and pedals as if the pressure increased the volume and tone. It was an intoxicating music that after a few moments came as if harnessed by the hands of the choir director who started the bass, tenor and contralto for the singing of the *Gloria*. The majesty of the Latin text, the solemn melody of the song, the vigor of the accompanying organ music has never left me and I think that the singing of the Easter *Gloria* constituted my musical imprinting. None of my family the past five generations had ever studied music. My dad hated any instrument or devilry (radio and turntable) that made sounds. Let's say that, as a boy, I just didn't live in an environment suitable for developing musical talent. But as happens with the DNA of humans with is continually strengthened thanks to the ability to regenerate and change obsolete genes for the survival of the species, so it must have also happened in my case. Instead of the genes for hunting in the forest and fighting ferocious beasts typical of cavemen, and perhaps my ancestors too, the music gene and the passion for musical instrument had developed in me.

We left school at 12:30. Before I got home, Vittorio and I went to church. Not because of an act of devotion, but because we had found out where the sacristan kept the organ keys. We sneaked into the sacristy and took the keys that allowed us to unlock the wooden gate of the magnificent organ. The view of the two rows of keyboards with all the various registers, from the harpsichord to the violin, for the oboe to the clarinet, enchanted us every time. And then there were the volume pedals, the pedal of the lowest notes, the foot switches for the tones, the reverb and the choral. It was a marvelous instrument with more than a thousand pipes — each ready to emit its specific sound in response to the organist's touch.

One day, we were trying to understand something by pressing the various keys and pedals that released unconnected sounds, when the furious archpriest came and slammed the cover on our hands and drove us away from the church. For a while, I had no chance to repeat my first experience as an aspiring musician, but three years later, as the music gene continued to print proteins and hormones in me, I bought a book for a method to learn how to play the piano from a used book market. I discovered a tempting world of eight and sixteenth notes, treble and bass clefs, pauses, rhythms, solfeggios (scales) and metronomes. But it was a theoretical world because there was no mention of instruments at my house. At Christmas however, I received a small accordion with a one and a half octave keyboard from the usual uncle Gigi. Twenty-five keys in all between black and white. To be able to play it with two hands like a harmonium or a piano, I nailed the keyboard on a table and solved the bellows problem by asking those who happened to be within range, especially my brother Gianni, to push the bellows back and forth. But since the volunteers for the bellows were scarce, I could hardly play, and my progress was poor. Then a turntable arrived at our house and I began to ask for a few organ records. I was struck by a 33rpm record of Albert Schweitzer who played Bach. Albert, as I called him, as an organist and doctor, immediately became my model. I was sure that one day I would become a doctor. I had it in my blood. To become an organist however, I had some doubts. It seemed to me that I was far behind on the roadmap.

An important turning point in my life as a musician occurred when my brother's girlfriend gave him a guitar. My brother wasn't too interested, so I immediately took it. The guitar was good, but I didn't know where to start. Tiziano, the brother of my future sister-in-law, played in a group from Vicenza called "The Gentlemen." When he came up to the Altopiano to visit us, I would seize him for a half hour of lessons. At twelve, I had learned some melody and some small solos and the guitarist of the complex "I Roversi" of Asiago had taught me a series of chords sufficient to accompany two or three songs. Those were the times of the new musical groups. A group from Liverpool had just launched *Please Please Me*. The Beatles were born, but surprisingly the name derived from cockroaches., and not as I had always wanted to think that their name could have been derived from beat-less (even if it had one less "s") or the ones without a heartbeat, since the heart of so many young girls stopped when Paul or George sang into the same microphone on stage. The Beatles really did leave you breathless. You couldn't help but try and emulate their songs to the delight of the four friends who would meet on Saturday afternoon festivities.

At the age of 14, I gave up all my savings — almost five thousand lire, and I bought a second-hand electric guitar. Together with Flavio and Enrico, we got a new amplifier. The two loudspeakers were made by us with horns mounted on large plywood boxes. We used my garage as a rehearsal room. We still needed a drummer. There weren't any in our village because the drum sets were too expensive, but we were still happy, and in the evenings, any excuse was a good excuse to play. We listened over and over to the 45 rpms of the Beatles and tried to reproduce their songs as true as possible. Meanwhile, I benefitted from the many long months I had spent learning sacred vocal music and practiced modulating my voice and was now capable of full falsetto. I was now capable of discreetly performing my first song *E la pioggia che va* from the Rokes, with music and words by Shel Shapiro. Shel had a famous red EKO guitar, characterized by two wings. I could hardly believe that he could follow his chords and sing with his Italian American accent that was so cool at the time. After a few months I had collected quite a few scores, most of which were purchased at the Ricordi Music store in Milan. I played for the sake of playing pieces I liked, but also because I soon understood that a guitar was as valuable as water in the desert during the summer in Jesolo. My songs were *Pooh's Piccola Katy*, *Un'Anima Pura* from the Rokes, *Io Ho in Mente Te* from Equipe 84 etc…

We would listen on Saturday afternoons to the radio program titled *Bandiera Gialla* and we would go so far as to compose songs based on the same title that Gianni Pettenati sang. If you only knew how many evenings we spent at the beach with the young people from our town. Back then, there were no families at the campsites, but only young people. Full busses of Swedish, Finnish and Dutch girls who couldn't wait to spend a romantic evening with us "Italians," a guitar and the sea! My repertoire expanded further to include a whole series of covers that was nothing more than the translations of popular American songs. Pregherò from *Stand by Me*, Sei già di un altro from *Don't Worry Baby* etc…

Upon returning from one of those holidays, on the eve of the beginning of the third year of high school, I found a group of friends from Vicenza that had made up a group that lacked a singer and solo guitar. In the meantime, with my savings I had now also bought a semi-acoustic EKO guitar. It wasn't a big deal but did its job in an honest manner. The group contacted me and we tried to play together in a basement similar to the one that I had always used to play. Eventually they asked me to join the group and we baptized it with a new name the "F-104," in honor of the missile shaped fighter recently supplied to the Italian Air Force and already called by those that piloted it: the "flying coffin." The theme song that the group used to open our concerts was composed by me and began with a long whistle that gradually increased in volume and ended abruptly with a loud drum beat to simulate the overcoming of the sound barrier. This was followed by a series of power chords, the two-note chords that are the foundation of modern rock. We had begun to play some evenings and at birthdays and graduation parties.

We were proud of our group, even though we were aware of our limitations. The group included Guido, the second guitarist — who had his own idea of rhythm; Luciano, the bass player and best looking of the group and whose girlfriend was glued to the amplifier every evening to defend her territory from occasional competitors; Bruno, the drummer, who often got lost in the middle of a passage and had to get to the end of the song to resume the rhythm; Nicola, the crazy keyboard player, who sometimes went off on some crazy solo that was absolutely out of nowhere. I guess you could say that I was the "least worst" of the group, and certainly not a star, but I sang well. I was driving the ensemble but wasn't a real conductor. It was clear that we would not go anywhere and that we had to capitalize on our small successes. We had a song called *Maybe Tomorrow*, that was particularly good for me and we played it five or six times per evening. Of course, I had some other workhorses like the Bee Gees — *I Started a Joke*, the Beatles' *Yesterday* and Procol Harum's *A Whiter Shade of Pale*. One evening was particularly embarrassing as we found ourselves playing for a British school party and more than half of our repertoire was in English. I sang by heart and admitting that I didn't know a word of English, had the feeling of being under scrutiny. But actually, the evening went well and in addition to the agreed-on amount of fifteen thousand lire, they also gave us food and a little extra compensation. On returning home from the International Hotel, my scooter broke down and I walked for more than seven kilometers at tow in the morning with a guitar on my shoulder pushing the damned Lambrettino scooter (but cursed the scooter only for that evening).

We reached the final test of high school — called "The Maturity Exam," that was followed by a fantastic vacation. We found an engagement in Jesolo, in an outdoor dance area by the Piazza Brescia. We received five thousand lire an evening plus food and lodging. The food was pretty good because the restaurant owner's wife treated us like her children. For the accommodation, instead, we had to settle for a room in a garage area that we shared among five of us. Luckily, we were also close to the maid's room, who was also our age.

Her name was Wilma. She arrived each evening about half past nine and came for ten evenings in a row. She brought a friend of hers and they listened to us, despite that our repertoire was not too varied. She was beautiful, tanned with black hair as smooth and light as silk. So breathtakingly beautiful. We locked eyes for every moment that I sang.

One evening, on the eleventh, she arrived and sat down at the usual table with her usual friend. Two boys with Milan accents also arrived and began to buzz around them. We decreed an impromptu break with a set that ended with the song Relax. Together with the bassist we went towards them. We hadn't even reached the table when she pointed her finger at me and said to the two "I am his girlfriend and the other is my cousin's boyfriend." The two boys from Milan left, disillusioned. From that moment, it was downhill from there. I spent the whole month playing and looking into her eyes and dancing with her in the moments of pause when we played recorded music to the "Semprini" voice-stereo system that we had rented. The "Montarbo" system would have been better, but the Semprini was an old system that we had from a famous group that sold it to us at a good price. I have to say that I was always grateful to "Mr. Semprini," when she told me that my voice was beautiful.

The magic of the guitar and the songs continued even after returning from vacation, until the Campedello concert. Campedello was a country town near Vicenza where we wanted to simulate the exploits of the grand Woodstock. Before the show I had been given a letter. I didn't open it immediately because I had to assemble and test the instrument and check the sounds. There were other groups — all very good, and we didn't want to cut a bad figure. I remember the letter so well, shortly before the performance. It was Wilma, who left me, not for lack of love, but because the light of our love would have been extinguished from the distance (she lived in Verona). "Like the light of the candle which after shining all night, becomes invisible at the first flashes of morning." I went to the stage and performed our three songs without feeling. Eventually, I took off my guitar and swore to myself that I would never play again until I found a love greater than what I had just lost.

***

True to my oath, I did return to the stage again with an electric guitar and a microphone in my hand in front of an audience exactly forty-five years later. For more than twelve years I was the head of the Nephrology department at the Vicenza Hospital and I had set up IRRIV with an extraordinary group of researchers. But research costs money and the fellows — although full of good will, needed to also live. For some time, I had been struggling to find the necessary funding for our cause. One day, Ciccio and Kecco, father and son, talented and full of heart musicians, tell me that their group is available for a charity show. They offered to help me by making available the most effective tool for reaching people's hearts — that of music. Wonderful. Knowing my musical background, they talk to me about their sixty's repertoire. We decided that the show would be called *"California Dreaming"* as the same name from the Mamas and Papas song. The mayor let us use the civic theater of Vicenza and from that moment, the operation of solidarity and friendships started which transformed into 900 places for the event. But something else also happened during the preparation. One evening at dinner, one week before the show, Ciccio and Kecco told me point-blank "Of course the show would have another flavor if you joined us and played and sang with the group." A twinkle in my eyes, thunder in my ears, lightning in my heart. I hadn't played or sang for years, but who cared. After all, I am a doctor, I thought. Nobody expects great things from a department head. If we do it for charity, the public would be lenient. So, I accepted facing a week of fear and excitement. I dusted off my old twelve string Gibson. I had bought it in New York in the year 2000, more as a memorabilia than as an instrument, because it was broken and I like to think that it had been damaged precisely in that Woodstock concert where the best musicians of our time had performed. I had it repaired. According to Kecco, it was an extraordinary instrument with beautiful harmonics. We planned the interlude that I would play with them. We would reproduce one of those 60's festivities that were organized on Saturday afternoons at friends' houses when the songs of the "Yellow Flag" were all sung together. The band would do some pieces to warm the environment, and then I would join in. It would be me and Ciccio sitting on two stools in front of the audience to open the various songs, while the band from behind would follow us in the second verse in a crescendo of choirs and sounds. Ciccio and Kecco actually had no idea what gift they were giving me — the joy of realizing the most beautiful dream of singing and playing with a real band. I will be forever grateful to them.

The curtain opened and the band began with E la pioggia che va, the very first song that I sang and played as a boy. My hands were sweating, and my heart raced. The moment had arrived! After Ciccio had finished un medley with the songs by Paul Anka, Kecco announced my entrance "Now, the time has come to bring one of our fellow musicians on the scene, who joins the group tonight and performs for the sake of his patients. He is the one who created the Vicenza Research Institute from scratch and a true master of research, the rock star "The Doc." I was greeted by thunderous and affectionate applause. We had done a one-off rehearsal the day before. I had the scores written on the computer, with a 36 character and a double spacing so they could be read from a distance. I didn't have time to memorize the chords, but the guys in the band were all with me, aware that their help will maybe not make me as good as them, but certainly, one of them. I sat on the stool next to Ciccio. Kecco handed me the guitar. My adrenaline was skyrocketing. I began with a greeting what was also a request for goodwill. "Being the head of a department like ours is complex. Being a researcher is a difficult job, being a musician is complicated. To do all three is a "vero casino" (which in Italian translates to a big mess)." The public broke out in laughter and I understood that the ice had been broken.

I had sworn to myself that I would never play or sing in public again until I had met a love greater than that for which I had stopped forty years ago. Today, I can easily say I have found at least three loves. The first is medicine — a mission of love; the second is that of research — a true passion and the third, but not least, is the one for the person who has always been at my side and lives with me the madness that I sometimes invent." And with my heart swollen with joy, I proudly play a "D-major" chord for *Hey Paola*, looking lovingly into my wife Paola's eyes. At first my voice was a little unsteady, but then it consolidated and became clear as the water that flowed from a source that had been closed for many years. "True love meaning planning a life for two, be together." The band followed me, and I understood that with them for this evening, I had gone far because this time they were the very good and I was the worst. The songs followed one after the other, with dialogue between Ciccio and me. "Do you remember this?" and "Remember this other one?" I sing *The Power of Love, Yesterday, the World, Blue Water, Clear Water, Oh Carol* and at a certain moment, the whole theater sang with me. People are happy and I am happy with them. Finally, with the help of the giant music scores printed in front of me, I rediscovered the language of angels that I thought I had forgotten.

The magic of ice

I WAS FOUR years old the day my father took me to the Millepini di Asiago and put on rudimentary skates that were strapped to my feet with an English wrench. He accompanied me to the middle of the ice field and said to me "skate." I consumed two pairs of heavy pants that year because the magic of ice consumed me, and I couldn't help but go every day all winter to the skating rink. The grown-ups would slide on the ice as if they were flying and the girls would dance and pirouette. I was looking forward to becoming as good as them and I applied myself with determination. Ever since that winter, I have always looked forward to the cold of December which would bring frost and I also hoped that the March sun would be late in order to prolong the skating season a little more.

At seven, I had my first pair of real "full boot" skates. They were beautiful. By now, I had learned to skate fairly well and I flew up and down the rink shooting and braking like a madman. On winter Sundays, the children of Asiago "Kinder Slegar," as referred to as the older people that spoke Cimbro called us, went to the Millepini to see the adults who played hockey against the teams of Agordo, Alleghe and Renon. It was a championship poor in resources but full of enthusiasm and cheering. The courage and impetus were extraordinary and there were often big fights when a referee would make an injudicious call for a foul and the players might think about restoring a little justice on the field. My friends and I would arrive at the Millepini quite early to make sure we could get the best seats made from piles of snow by the ring without caring for the inexorably iced feet. Those positions were also ideal to pick up any broken sticks that players had thrown from the rink. That was actually how I built my first hockey stick. I retrieved a stick with a broken head and was aided by a friendly carpenter. I fixed it by adding a new spatula made from scrap board from the nearby FADA, a furniture factory that has now disappeared. I was not the only one among friends to have had that chance, and with these improvised pieces of equipment, we started our hockey activity on the ponds used to provide drinking water for cows in the summer. When the ice melted, the corridor at the bottom of the stairs was also a good alternative to continue our games. If you only knew how many windows we broke and how many slaps were incurred when we would dent a door with the wooden disc recuperated from a beech tree trunk.

One day my godfather, who ran a bookstore, gave me a book on hockey rules that described so many new and interesting things. I adored that book and guarded it as a treasure. I kept it under the pillow on my bed and leafed through it every chance I had, but especially before falling to sleep. Sleep sometimes overcame me and carried these stories into my dreams where I imagined myself to be a real player with a team of players ready to face opponents. The dream of ice skating has been one of the recurring dreams of my life. Even today, sometimes I dream of flying down the ice with skates and a hockey stick. I always wake up happy after that.

One day, my dream became a reality when at the age of eleven I jointed the student team. Our equipment consisted of a series of protections derived from things handed down from the adult team. A jumble of frayed gloves, shin guards, sweaters with more holes than actual wool which might even be risky on the ice, but it was "our" uniform because it had the yellow and red colors of the municipal flag that Asiago had always used for the first team. We did a bit of training in the evenings around half past six, after homework and at the end of the working day for the older ones. The whole practice didn't last much more than an hour as I had to always be home by half past seven, sitting at the table for dinner. My father would never compromise on this. Sometimes crammed into the van of the electrician from Asiago, we went away to a nearby town for a game with a rival team. They were moments of great happiness for me. Life and dreams merged into the magic of ice. Those who have not lived in the Altopiano can't understand the passion for this sport that enters your heart and holds your soul ransom. Hockey is not only elegant, but very fast and athletic. So much that there is not one player who doesn't have a permanent face scar or replaced teeth. The ritual of the call to the first ice and the evenings at the Millepini to play with friends, the games of the adult teams, the dream of a full stick and decent equipment continued for three seasons until it was time for me to go to college. My playing career stopped at thirteen, when not only did they not send me to the summer internship in Cortina, which was the dream of all of us kids, but they asked me to return the "equipment" as I returned to Asiago on a Saturday for a few hours. I think it was one of the biggest disappointments and most suffered moments of my life. I left the team. My personal joy of running on sharp blades towards the goal would never be there again. My ambitions that lay ahead of me, were left only in my dreams. For all the years of gymnasium and high school, for those of the university and throughout my life as a doctor and researcher, the passion for hockey has never left me.

I went to see some of the Asiago games that arrived in the A Series with both joy and sadness, while I watched the boys of the under 16 team, the team in which I was supposed to be a soldier. They now had brand new and perfect equipment, as were gloves, trousers and sweaters. I still have a slightly creased photo of my old team that I keep in my wallet.

Exactly fifty years have passed since I had returned my skates and hockey sticks. I have since become a mature person with a long career as a doctor and research on my shoulders, but I continue to hold Asiago in my heart and never ceased to help anyone from there in need, as if the mission of my father the old general practitioner continued to also be my calling. In mid-November, I received a letter from the mayor, the son of our historic captain Cesare Gios, and he informed me that the city of Asiago had decided to grant me honorary citizenship. The delivery of the diploma, the first in the history of the town administration, would take place at the town hall in early December. On the same day, the friends of Asiago informed me that to solemnize the event, they organized a friendly hockey match between the A Series team and that of the "Old Glories," the legendary "Old Bears," I.e., the player who had played in that first team and that formed their own group to continue playing in a friendly and buoyant manner at least once a week. I received an SMS from Fabrizio, known as Cin (in Asiago, everyone has a nickname because there are hundreds of people with the same surname). He asked if I would like to launch the puck at the beginning of the game. This is an honor usually only reserved for the great champions of the past, and I am not (only in my dreams). Suddenly remembering the rock concert with the Ciccio Corona band, a crazy idea flashed into my mind. "Cin," I said on the phone, "What if I tried to skate with you? After all, it is a friendly match and with expert players there is no risk of getting hurt. I could finally crown a dream and return for a moment to that boy who left his dream on the ice of Asiago."

"Doctor," Cin replies, "you are completely crazy" but after a moment, "but why not?"

The rumor spread and a competition was created among the Old Bears to give me what I needed to play. One gave me the shin guards, another the back and another the shell. All the precious pieces to protect the family jewels. "Il Falco," Lucio Topatigh, perhaps the greatest Italian Hockey player of all time gave me the skates and sticks. I hadn't worn skates for more than fifty years, and in the meantime, hadn't even practiced sports or gone to the gym on a regular basis. I had to widen the trousers a little, because I couldn't compress my stomach too much. We decided to test the Monday before the official game. Cin, with a gesture of great affection, gave me his shirt. "Doc" he tells me in the locker room "Real Madrid has the CR7, Cristiano Ronaldo, you will be our CR19." Nineteen has always been an important number in my life and will be once again. The test shows all my limitations, but it doesn't matter. Everyone encourages me and in any case, they think that once the game of life is over — as we called it- I will go back to being a doctor and a researcher, keeping a good memory of the evening and nothing more. They don't know how wrong they are. Once I have found the ice route again, I think to myself, I will never lose it again. But for the moment I have other things to think about; being able to stand up, trying to hit the puck and avoid hurting myself. In the first test before the match, I must have set in motion muscles that had not been used for years, because the following week, I as literally paralyzed with pain. There was no part of my body that didn't hurt, but my adrenaline was sky high and the only physical problem I feel is that of being able to stay inside my own skin. I am so excited that in one night I write a booklet entitled "Ice." It is a little book of a little more than a hundred pages, that my friend Giancarlo of the Busato print shop manages to put together in three days, in time for the game.

Everything is ready. The day has come and the excitement of receiving from band with the seal of the great city of Asiago is very great. I think of my father and tell myself that this honor is largely dedicated to him. Some senior city councilors still remembered him as the town doctor, a generous man. While I am signing some books for those present, Ciano, the goalkeeper of the Old Bears gestures to me indicating the clock. It is time to climb the Millepini like the old days, but this time with a shiny new bag full of protections and almost new equipment.

They welcomed me when I entered the crowded locker room with a cry "come on CR19!." Gaetano presented me with a stick that had been signed by everyone. John John took the new shirts out of the box and officially gave me the shirt with the number 19 and printed with my name in large letters. I felt such emotion that was even more intense than when I had received the Lifetime Achievement Award for the best researcher of the year or as an honorary member of the American Society of Nephrology. We began to dress, and I started getting advice. "First the breeches and then the skates. Put a band inside your helmet for sweat. Tighten the shin guards with tape. Put a little soap or wax on the stick tape to prevent the snow from sticking." I hear this, but in a surreal manner. I am in a trance. I can hardly believe this is all happening. I enter the field moving my skates with some uncertainty and look for Paola. She speaks to me with her eyes as if to say "go champion, you have desired this your whole life. Don't miss a moment of the immense joy." The mayor Andrea had taken off the Italian tricolor band and had replaced it with a shirt bearing the number 4 that had been his father's and makes me feel close. Topa with his legendary 27 gives me some advice to avoid making a bad figure. They were all there: Gigi, Majo, Bericus, John John, Cape and of course Cin. We did some warm ups, then off we went. The referee was someone I used to know, Francesco from Camporovere who had played at the same time as me, but then became a national referee. The stands were full of people cheerful and curious. Maybe some consider me a little crazy, but now I am their fellow citizen, so there I am. The game begins. The engagement is with the front line and I finally find myself in the role of center that I had left hanging fifty years earlier. The A Series team plays relaxed, but not too much because they also don't want to make a bad impression. Topa, still makes them turn and forces them to defend themselves. At a certain moment they make a bad body check and the referee declares "rigore" (a penalty shot). "You have to make it!" they say almost in chorus. I realize that they still really cared for me and wanted to give me the opportunity to enjoy this moment to the fullest. Cin came close to me and suggested that I aim between the goalkeeper's legs ten centimeters high. What advice! I start from the center, make an English pass to the right to arrive just in front of the goalkeeper with the left loaded. I take my aim as Cin suggested and Wham! A goal! The stadium exploded. Gloves and helmets were thrown onto the ice. I ran to beat the glove of my companions. I really don't know if I was really so good at putting the puck in the right place, or if the goalkeeper was better at letting the shot pass. But actually — who cares. It doesn't matter. It was a feast of friendship and sport. We were not there to win, but to play and we all won the game of life that evening, and in particular for me, it was a dream come true. I was never so happy. The joy remained in my heart together with an immense satisfaction. A sort of appointment with destiny and with ice, missed fifty years earlier and found in mature age, but with equal if not greater enthusiasm.

Five years have passed since that fantastic day and the memory still lives inside me as though it were yesterday. Those who thought I would give up after that repatriation are still surprised. If they are not traveling around the world, they would see me return to the Millepini every Monday evening. It is like a ritual. At seven, after twelve hours at the hospital, I get in the car and go to the Altopiano. At each turn going up the Costo road, I feel my mind clear. When I arrive at Barricata, and then Campiello, I am completely free and happy. When I finally arrive in the locker room around 8:00 p.m., I usually only find Cyan, who, like me loves to arrive early to enjoy a moment of peace. The incredible stench emanating from every hockey dressing room seems to me like a mountain perfume that I inhale like a balsam. My bag is always full of equipment, always shining, because since my passion became know in the public domain, I often receive special gifts from Canada or the United States. A new helmet with the number 19, a shirt from the Pittsburgh Penguins or Toronto Maple Leafs. We talk a little more and fill a bucket full of snow to hold a bottle of prosecco for the traditional toast after the game. A third time with bread, salami, mountain cheese and Berico desserts.

We start to get dressed. These are the first calm moments of my day. Slowly the others arrive. Sometimes they will also show me the results of the exams of their mother or brother in law, or we will have a makeshift medical study for consulting or diagnoses. Everyone tells me about events that happened during the week and ask me about my adventures. Where did I go, did I have photos of the far away airports. "Do you know Doc" said Cin, "we all thought you would have abandoned the group after that first great game. No one thought you would have had the perseverance to continue and try to improve with a lot of effort." So jokingly, I tell them that I have an advantage over them because I will continue to improve while they can only get worse. Received by endless laughter. Carefree and pure soulmates. I found real friends in those guys. Almost a family. At the beginning they accepted me because I was the important professor. Today, they see me as their friend and that's it. One who has the same passion for hockey, only that I need to stop for other activities for a while. At the end of the warm-up we do the usual white against red game and the gag is that whites always win, even when the reds win. The goal abacus is broken and does not count how many goals are scored, but rather we keep track of how many good moments we spend on the ice.

From that first time, we have continued to play with the players from the A series every year. They are now in the higher levels of Italian hockey having won the league titles and Alpe league championships. Sometimes on the field we even kidnap the captain "Strice," and dress him in our shirts. Other times, we grabbed players from the other team and kept them stuck in the balustrade. It is a nice game that makes the public understand the importance of sport to help the weakest. We do this to greet blood donors as heroes. We do it to give new hope to our patients by collecting some money for research. We do it so that everyone can win at the game of life. At the awards, the two cups are strictly the same because there are always two winners and no losers. After all, Piercarlo, the president of the Asiago 1935 Hockey club and I have two teams to lead to victory. For him, it is a league title in the highest division, for me concrete results in medical research. We have fantastic players and the game is an opportunity to introduce them to people.

A couple of years ago, it was decided to withdraw Topa's shirt, which is an extraordinary honor for a player, because it means that nobody after him will have his number. That honor was to be given to Lucio Topatigh during the European Championships and on that occasion he needed to give his speech in English. Falco approached me and said, "Ciao Doc, I am only so-so at English, can you give me a hand?" I felt honored that he asked me, so I diligently applied myself to writing down some appropriate thoughts. The result was a simple but heartfelt speech that he read with the right warmth at the time of the award ceremony and was then uploaded on YouTube.

"Although hockey is not a widespread sport in Italy, it is in the hearts of many people, especially in our northern regions. Having devoted a lot of time and energy to this sport and therefore knowing it well, I consider it an instrument of redemption, happiness and interaction with other human beings. Hockey is also a bridge between new generations and past generations in a continuum of friendship and commitment. Playing hockey isn't just about exercising or competing for a game win. Playing hockey means belonging to a team, being a friend with friends, is to commit to a lifestyle made of principles, honor and sacrifice. We can all be champions. Every player who has these feelings is a champion regardless of the goals scored or the technique acquired on the pitch."

I was happy and proud to hear that speech, thinking that the words that came out of the mouth of that unreachable champion, and that he had made his own, had first come from the heart of an "adopted" simple center player of the Old bears: the enthusiastic apprentice champion CR19.

Festina lente (Hurry Slowly)

WHAT IS the right pace of life? I still don't know. Everyone has his measure. I would have always been for a peaceful life, but today I find myself living at a speed that many friends and my wife define as crazy. I am caught up in a whirlwind of commitments, of projects to be carried out quickly, of frantic and long journeys for which time is never enough. I realize that it may seem crazy to come and go to Australia in three days with the difficulties of traveling and changing the rhythm of life, the environment and the time zone. But I made a virtue of necessity and, especially after the collapse of the Twin Towers, planning travel has become extremely difficult. I have become an astute traveler. To survive the inconvenience that a frequent traveler like me encounters, I have developed a series of expertise and techniques that allows me to avoid delays, hitches, loose connections or remain prisoner in a terminal for hours like Tom Hanks in the film of the same name.

My first trick lies in the preparation of my baggage. I limit myself strictly to hand luggage. This streamlines complex passages to customs, avoids delays in the delivery and the loss of personal effects in the event of a tight missed connection. Of course, hand luggage, has its drawbacks: limited weight and volume. But does that really matter? Now my travels, even when I go to the other sider of the world lasts for a maximum of four days: three shirts, a few changes of underwear, a small bag for carrying medicine (not boxes), toiletries and shaving supplies (all in miniature versions). No scissors or other possibly prohibited items to avoid their confiscation. If I want to bring a bottle of wine to a friend across the ocean, I buy this at the duty-free store at my last connection. Usually, I am OK to just bring a small cabin trolley, that meets the requirements for all the airlines, that I see are being sometimes rigorously controlled — particularly for the low-cost carriers. For the choice of flying from Vicenza to the boarding airport, I take into account the variables that can influence traffic. In Venice in the summer, the autopark garage for the Marco Polo Airport is blocked by weekend tourists who go to the beach. In Verona, mobility goes haywire every time there is a fair, especially for Vinitaly. On the Ostiense, the traffic is chaotic when hordes of vacationers from Rome head to the shores, as well as during the peak hours each day. In large metropolitan areas with multiple airports, I play close attention to my landing details. Once, I was flying to Sao Paulo and I had not noticed that I would be landing at the International terminal, while my connection was leaving from Congojas. It took me three hours by car to go from one airport to the other. But in the end, the delay hadn't made a difference because my connection had been canceled due to bankruptcy and the final shutdown of the Varig company. A hundred-dollar tip to an employee behind the counter, pressed by a row of wild stranded passengers, allowed me on that occasion to find a flight to Gramado with Lan Chile. In Rome, as in Brussels, on Thursdays and Fridays are the days when politicians return home so I absolutely avoid arriving late to check in because there is a high probability that they might have resold my place leaving me stranded. My habit now is to check-in online, well in advance and ensuring that my boarding pass is with me in time. Queues are a problem, but I've learned to get around them. When I arrive at a big airport, like Frankfurt, I sometimes leave the terminal and return later, rather than joining the long line waiting for the numerous connecting flights (there is hardly anyone in the evening). If I allow myself a nap in the waiting room, I sleep with an ear attentive to the announcements and I often look at the flight board. Changes of gates, cancellations or delays will not catch me unprepared. Over time and flying a lot, I have learned to recognize the various airports by also their smells. In Seoul, as in many other ports of the Orient, you can smell the classic aroma of garlic everywhere. In Marrakech, the rooms smell of spices, while in Bangkok you can perceive a scent of orchids and frangipani. Each also has some specialty that makes the "environment." In Buenos Aires, there is the fabulous grilled provolone seasoned with tomato and oregano, while in the corridor C of the Rio airport there is a really excellent churrascheria. In Frankfurt, there is a baker offering the best pretzels, and if I arrive in the evening, I take them home for dinner. If you are in hurry to go through security, you need to keep in mind that the more communist the country, the more "the VIP status" works. In China or Iran, they do not accept the definition of Very Important Person (VIP) contrary to their "democratic" principals and their history, but if you are a CIP (Commercially Interesting Person), It is fine and you have preferential lanes for business and first class. In America, if you are lucky enough to be labeled as pre-TSA (Transportation Security Administration), you don't even have to take your computer out of the bag. I have also learned to collect all the cards of companies that can be found, because for the moment, a "frequent traveler" status can be discriminating. It can allow you to get priority on a waiting list or access to a private room. Upon boarding, I position myself in time at the gate to be among the first to go up in order to find space for hand luggage and to choose a place in the aisle to be free to move and at the end of the flight, ready to go in case of tight connections or delays. On long trips, I try to reduce variables that could create anxiety by adopting small tricks, such as putting the phone, wallet, passport and tickets (I.e., the fundamentals of the traveler) always in the same place, so as to make sure that they are all within easy reach. I take a lot of liquids to keep myself hydrated. I avoid being enticed by tasty but heavy menus. I abandon myself to restful sleep as soon as conditions allow and when I arrive, I enter energy saving mode, leaving aside any ambition of environmental or cultural tourism. If I can, I also avoid social dinners and any kind of distraction that does not affect the duties of courtesy towards the people that host me. I make sure that the stop at the destination is as short as possible to avoid the consequences of the time zone change on the return. I spend most of my time in the bedroom sleeping or working on the computer. This allows me to return to the ward and resume work almost as though I had never left.

I agree that my method is not a particularly exciting way to travel, but it is efficient. After all this is the beauty and ugliness of being a true citizen of the world.

But every once in a while, I also unplug, as they say, and return to a slowed down world, that of my mountains, which seem to me to be the same as when I lived there as a child, and from which I regularly draw serenity and peace. The opportunity I never miss is that of the Grande Rogazione. It is a votive procession that the inhabitants of the Asiago Altopiano have been repeating for hundreds of years in thanksgiving to God for the cessation of a long plague. The Rogazione runs for thirty-six kilometers with stages in the capitals of the Altopiano and has a lot of participation, particularly in this third millennium. It remains a staple in the heart of every inhabitant of Asiago. I believe I have participated in every edition from since I was four years old. How many memories! The never-ending advice and admonishments of the days prior to the event were: "Do you have the right shoes? Because you know, in the first stretch across the field you will get your feet wet. Are you sure you have enough sandwiches in the bag, did you get your windbreaker?" But we didn't worry too much because we knew that every tactical error would be corrected at the first stop at the Lazzaretto where friends and relatives, waiting for mass and a picnic, supplied us with sweaters and food. It was an expected and anticipated stop, also because here the girls showed their crushes and preferences by giving eggs painted with the flowers and herbs of the meadows to the boys. The boys hoarded these and made comparisons with the others because from the number and care with which they had been packaged, you could understand your net worth to the girls. Each boy then had to keep in mind the physiognomies of the donors because the girls expected a reciprocal gift of the "cuco," a terracotta flute, at the "Festa del ciclamino di Cesuna."

The annual procession of the Grande Rogazione opened with a flag and a cross. Don Enrico Barbiero, the priest, who was the only one who completed a part of the journey on the back of a mule. The crowd of the highlands followed him chanting orderly. I remember the pride with which the boys passed from one year to the other from the youth sector to the adult section. Toni said to us, "Stay here kids, but sing the litanies with us all day." And it was exciting to repeat aloud in the woods, with the spirit of prayer and the mountain, the names of all the saints on the calendar. And how much to shout before Mount Catz! "I'll make it?" "Of course you will! If not we will help you!" the adults told me. And then all together to the top where we could then enjoy refreshments made above all for sharing. The last stop was in the Gallio forest in search of green branches that we would cut with our knives that had been sharpened before departure, to adorn the hair and mountain bags in the fashionable Cimbra style.

At the time of entry into Asiago, the songs multiplied and alternated between groups of men and women, boys and girls, proud to have completed the entire Rogazione process once again. We would go home exhausted. Once in bed, I anxiously called my mother and told her I still heard singing. "Don't worry" she said, "you are just tired, and the songs are still in your head."

I still love the Grande Rogazione as I did then. At the end of the procession and the day, we all feel happier and a little better. We say goodbye to friends with a "see you later in the square," but everyone knows in his heart that after a hot bath, he will prefer to stay at home and once in bed, to hear the songs of the litanies again in his head. Every year is like this and I don't want it to change because on that day, my life slows down and my world expands. It is a bit like the concept expressed by Einstein in the theory of relativity for which the speed of light is the limit value. The more you accelerate and get closer to that speed; the more time and space tend to contract. The further you move away and slow down the more time and space expand, precisely relatively.

Festina Lente — or *hurry slowly*, said the Latins. It was a phrase that the professor of the medical clinic often repeated to us when making a difficult diagnosis or evaluating a patient's condition. As doctors, we live at the side of the patient's beds in a perennial state of emergency for the desire to relieve the patient from physical ailments and, if possible, also from those of the soul. "A caress is worth more than a needle prick," my father used to repeat. The rhythms of the performances become faster and faster and our time together with the space around us, becomes infinitely small. Once upon a time an important event happened every six months. Today, three happen every day. The Pope's visit to our hospital for example, had been the event of a decade and for years there had been no talk of anything else. Instead the surreal crowding of events and problems that occurred in my department a few weeks ago. On the same day we had the first incompatible donor transplant, we also treated a patient with an innovative extracorporeal lifesaving technique after the cardiac surgeon conducted a heart valve repair intervention with a new minimally invasive technique. At the same time, we had to face the inspection of a quality certifier. The following day, I intervened at the inauguration of the new dialysis center of the Valdagno hospital in the morning, and that same evening left for China. It was Thursday, but already on Sunday I was back and returned to the ward Monday and found myself immersed in moments of ordinary frenzy. A colleague informed me that his mother had been hospitalized in intensive care. The Secretary informed me that two resigned to go to a different hospital and we were now short on staff. A biologist told me she was pregnant (fortunately planned) and that she would be absent for a year. At ten o'clock, the dialysis water production failed, while the hospital's data control center urges the approval of the budget sheet. At eleven o'clock, I have to settle an issue between a patient's family member and the patient's transport manager. At noon the commission for hospital infections proposes to isolate some patients in a ward which I consider unsuitable. At one o'clock, I am finally ready to have a bite to eat, but the computer system stops working and there is a stop for treatment prescriptions. In the meantime, a fistula operation in the operating room requires my presence. All of these are seasoned with an almost continuous interruption from collaborators who ask me for the classic "two minutes of attention." At 2 o'clock, I preside over a meeting with patients of the ward for an epicrisis of difficult cases and immediately afterwards, I must intervene at the meeting for AIDO, the Organ Donor Association. At 7 p.m. I finally can sit at the desk and complete a neglected work and think back to events of the past day. I had only come back from China last night, but seriously, who has time to afford a bit of time zone mind-blur? Someone will say that this is no longer a medical life. Sure, but it's okay if I can at least create the conditions for my collaborators and other doctors to work in a tranquil manner. Doing it yourself is now almost impossible. The only solution is to delegate. If the school is good and the team is good, there will be no problem. *Festina lente*. In this type of life, as I said, one must occasionally unplug and take a break. And since the Grande Rogazione comes only once a year, I invented with my wife, another essential break: the appointment with the Camino de Santiago. For years, we have been planning a week in the north of Spain to walk the journey for 30 km a day for six continuous days. Jean de Pied de Port leads to Santiago de Compostela and then to Finisterre. We are not driven by a particular devotion, but by the desire to slow down to expand our space and take a path of simplicity and spirituality.

From Roncesvalles, we go down to a shady stream with a moderately packed and not too heavy backpack. We arrive in Pamplona when the echoes of the feast of San Firmino have just diminished. We continue towards Rioja, the wine region, where among the expanses of vines planted on the rocky bottom, the ritual of "comida" as the Spaniards say, that is moments of particular conviviality and friendship. Between Logrogno and Santo Domingo de la Calzada the path is flat with frequent taverns and inns. Señora Maria del Carmen is tired and does not want to cook for us, "but if you want" she tells us, "the potatoes and eggs are there and you can get by. I prepare a tortilla, that is a large omelet with potatoes. We eat it drinking the tinto Verano, a mix of wine with low alcohol content and soft drinks which reminds me of certain drinks from my Altopiano. It's fantastic with ice. They guys we meet in the Camino all have happy faces, despite the blisters on their feet. Passing from the Castilla y Leon and stopping in the Paradores of Burgos and Leon, we are enchanted by the splendor of classic architecture. But to the big cities, we prefer the "mar de Castilla," the incredible sight of the wheat fields that sway in the wind like waves of a golden sea. The sky is blue, and the soul is free. The last hundred kilometers from

Sarria to Santiago are the culmination of the long journey. When you finally arrive and can put your feet on the seal of Santiago, together with the other many pilgrims, there is the taste of redemption and victory, even if in this journey, walking and the path are much more important than the goal itself. You end up with tired legs, but a clear mind. In Finisterre, we throw the "concha," the shell of St. James that accompanied us all the way, in the ocean as a sign of thanksgiving to nature and life. For every journey a shell, for every arrival in Campostela an emotion and the desire to start again with the serenity that this "slowing down of life" has always given us. Festina lente.

Then the moments of fury return. There are months in which, for every day spent in hospital to manage patients and staff, to quell conflicts, to experience enthusiasm, disappointments, disease, joys for new births and pains for affectionate patients who leave, I spend another on the plane or in congress centers and foreign universities to lecture in classrooms crammed with students. This is also "frenetic" as Americans would say. A frenetic succession of ups and downs. We must be able to have the strength to tell a patient about his painful destiny of illness and immediately afterwards give a smile to a transplant patient who returns to see life in color. We must live with the loss of people that you have followed over the months and years and with the need to continue to instill hope and desire to live in many others. So here is a third way to slow down my time and expand my world: raise the sail and to sea. I learned this from my friend Giancarlo when he convinced me to get on his boat for the first time. A mountaineer like me on a plastic shell beaten by the wind? I thought I would suffer and hate the narrow and cramped space of the hull — but no. On the boat, space is infinite because time sailing almost reduces to zero. Everything slows down, and the important thing is not to arrive but to go and navigate. Glide on the water in silence, without contact with the rest of the world. A day on a sailboat is like a month spent in the real world. The feeling of peace that the sea gives you and the rustling wind compensates for so many disappointments and bitterness, and even greater comfort, gives you friendship. The boat in fact, either cements or breaks friendships. With Giancarlo on the boat, we built a friendship of reinforced concrete.

Shangri-La

AFTER A TASTY MEAL of "pasta e fagioli" (pasta with beans) and a delicate grilled sea bass, we are conversing amiably waiting for dessert. It is the eve of the Epiphany, and we are at the Trattoria da Benetti at Costabissara for a dinner with some close friends. My wife had given Camilla, the youngest of Francesca's daughter, a set of colored crayons and zoomorphic stamps that she immediately put to work. She drew a big cat and called him Claudio, as indicated by the comment that came out of its mouth. Proud of her little masterpiece, she came to show it to me when my cell phone rang "Hello! Hello Claudio. son el Tata" «Eh, sento ben! Ma come mai a 'sta ora?» «A te telefono parché el bepin, piantando on ciodo 'nte la baràca, l'è cascà da la scala e i l'à portà in te l'ospedale de Vicensa. bisognaria ca te ghe dessi on ocio." «Ma, Tata, xe le diexe e meza de sera, xe sabo e son fora a sena». «sì, sì, ben. Ma someia ch'el se sia tutto roto drento, e chì nessun sa gnente. Vùto ca te passa so fradélo?." «no Tata. Prima ciamo l'ospedale e dopo te farò savere». «Ok, màndame un dispacio." (The conversation in a very local dialect with a lot of idiomatic sentences and words can be summarized as follows: "I am

Tata." "I hear you, but why a call at this time of the day?" " I call you because Beppino has fallen from the staircase and he was transferred to the hospital in Vicenza. It seems badly hurt. We would like you to visit him." But Tata, I am out for dinner, far from the hospital." "Yeah I know but he has multiple fractures, do you want to talk to his brother?." "Ok Tata, I will call the hospital and I will let you know").

I tried to summarize this short conversation to my friends, some from Milan, and they are intrigued. I have to explain that Tata, whose father was very close to my father, is the manager of the restaurant in Asiago where we go to eat pizza after the weekly hockey match with Cin, Majo and John John. Tata, just as many others, feels authorized to consult me at any time on any health problem that affects them, their relatives and their friends. Indeed, everyone in Asiago, for the simple fact of knowing me, finds it absolutely normal to call me outside or inside the hospital and to ask me for a consultation or help. One time it happened that someone asked the switchboard in Vicenza to be able to speak with "Claudio," and once the switchboard has realized that the Claudio sought by the "Asiaghese" is the head of the nephrology department, they pass the call. The caller asks me for an appointment because a specialist in Padova has made the diagnosis of a severe hernia. I try and explain that as a nephrologist, I really don't have anything to do with hernias, nor a bad tooth or foot pain. I was cut short "OK, I understand, but if you could just see me I would feel a little better." So understanding that I couldn't say "no" to one of my Asiago friends, I look at my agenda and suggest in dialect "OK, come in tomorrow morning" with the reply "No, sorry, I can't. I am hunting." "OK let's do Friday, okay for Friday, but not Friday morning as I have things to do in Asiago, better in the afternoon — do you agree." "OK, OK, I agree.

I go to Asiago with greater assiduity in the autumn months after the Epiphany when, free from tourists who bring urban customs and habits, the town returns to the Asiaghese. Some time ago after the Christmas holidays and while walking alone on a narrow street, I had stopped to look at a puddle of frozen water, when someone came up to me and said «La xe la possa del Marogna, dove i putei, ma anche qualchedun cressù, zugava a hockey». «E sì — gli dico —, me ricordo, parché ghe zugavo anca mi». «Ma alora, lu, xelo el dotor? Quelo che zuga a hockey?» «sì, mi son el dotor che zuga a hockey." «ben, che belo! Mi so che me papà xe sta salvà da so papà. El gaveva tanto mal de pansa, ma tanto, che i ga dovesto portarlo in ospedale. Alora so papà l'è andà dal chirurgo e el ghe ga dito: "Varda che te ghe da tajar da qua a qua, e no là." El chirurgo gavea in mente 'na roba, so papà n'altra, e gavea rason so papà. ben, ben. El vegna drento a bevare on giosso. E za che l'è qua, ghe tiro fora i esami che i me ga trovà el diabete." (translated from dialect into English this sounds approximately like this: " It is the frozen pond where we used to play hockey when we were kids. But.. But… are you the doctor? The one who still plays hockey? I know your father knew my father and saved his life taking him to the surgeon and giving directions on how to do the right surgery. Your father was right and he saved my father's life. Come in and seat down, while we drink a glass of wine I will show you my lab results. I am diabetic and I want to hear your opinion.")

When I am in Asiago, I am no longer Claudio Ronco, the nephrologist-physician-researcher- scientist, I am more than anything, the son of my father, the son of the town general doctor, with full authority and respect. Therefore, like him, I am on duty 24/7 and available to all: husbands, wives and children. In Asiago, couples made up of a true asiaghese (a man from Asiago) and an "outsider" are frequent. Indeed the unacknowledged dream of every Asiago merchant is to marry a lady from a different town with no local friends so she can stay in the shop and he can continue to carry on in the Asiago way — that is, go to the square, meet friends at the bar, go hunting, skiing and playing cards. Usually the "outsider" doesn't have the same confidence with me as her husband and if she needs something for her children, she starts with a hesitant request,"So Doctor, I don't know if I can ask this, I don't want to disturb you and sorry if…"and she continues full of cautions until he arrives inside the room "hey — Hello Claudio! Is it done? I am happy. Now we will drink some Prosecco."

And so it is with everyone, not only with those of my age or older. Even their grandchildren call me like you were their uncle. Because if things outside Asiago change with a geometric progression, on the Altopiano, they change with half an arithmetic progression. Those who chose to stay and live in Asiago remain in the village dimension of fifty years ago, and even the young people consider me part of their world and their affection. The Asiaghesi certainly respect me professionally, but they see me in the same light that they saw my father, the general practitioner that could cure the patient, and not just the illness. I remember one Christmas eve that my father brought me to a patient's house. He was in bad pain and knew he couldn't live and didn't want to live anymore. He brought him a panettone (Christmas cake) and sat with him talking the entire afternoon until he saw that his serenity had returned. And as they did with my dad who often called to settle family matters, so every now and then, someone who had an angry wife and possibly a bad conscience for some action would telephone me «Ciò, Claudio, quando ca-te-pol, fa na ciàcola con me mojère, che se no la me fa diventar mato; dighe ti che…» (Hey Claudio, when you can, please talk to my wife otherwise she will make me crazy, tell her that…). They saw the medical profession of the doctor in the right dimension. For them it is still a mission and for this reason it is free or almost free. In fact, none of those who stop me on the street and perhaps ask me to provide an urgent pediatric visit to their child, or bring me their analyses in the square to interpret, ever ask if they owe me anything. And that's fine with me, because in this way, I feel part of a simple genuine world, where the relationships that concern me are not determined by interests and calculations. We have a type of barter friendship. If I go to the butcher to buy a steak or at the bar in Bermi for a spritz, I can never pay. In fact, I have to take the spritz from time to time in different bars just to avoid that some manager's friend is offended.

Today, that humanization of medicine is included in the department's budget objectives. I am grateful to the Asiaghesi because they have been able to preserve a world made of human relationships, sometimes brusque and raw, but since, simple and direct; to which they have admitted me and where I restore myself as a man and where in some respects I play the role of the country doctor who maybe I would have like to have been if I had nine other lives to live.

For me to climb the Altopiano is always a cleansing experience. When I arrive at Treschè Conca, I often take the back secondary streets and stop for a few minutes to admire a large tree that surely is hundreds of years old. From that point, during the time of my childhood, two brothers, "the Bonomo brothers" were famous for their pre-war photo archive of Asiago, with the Altopiano seen from the west. One of the two, Renato, with his wife Ninetta lived in a house that had a common wall and balcony on the back of the house. The couple didn't have children and were always cheerful and welcoming. Surely they are some of the mildest people I have ever met. The other brother and the oldest, Ruggero, had married a nice lady, Athena. She was one of the first female graduates in mathematics with the legendary professor Zwirner in Padua. Renato and Ruggero ran the family business, which was a stationery, photo studio and print shop. You had to take them in small doses however and only if you had a lot of time. They were so meticulous that even if they needed to give an inexpensive one lira sheet of paper to a schoolboy, they would make every other paying customer wait. Tourists far preferred to deal with Ninetta, who had a dynamic character and who could revolutionize the shop in just an afternoon, changing it to meet the decorations for every season. Every evening Renato and Ninetta went to the railing of the shared balcony to play cards with us and watch the first television programs on our small 14 inch Telfunken TV. When my parents would go away for a day or two, they welcomed me into their home like a son, made me do my homework and in the evening they would put me to sleep in the bedroom at the end of the hallway with "grandma Vittoria" Ninetta's mother. In this way, over time, they became my Uncle Renato and my Aunt Ninetta, and their stationery shop became my home. The opportunity to do something different with Uncle Renato came four times a year, when the Bonomo brothers left with weapons and luggage and went to "take pictures" from which to obtain postcards to sell in their shop. They were shots that were carefully studied and patiently planned for days or even weeks in order to capture just the right shine of the snow, the iridescent color of the foliage, the tender green of the pine cones, the fresh clearness of the landscape after a summer storm.

"You see" said Uncle Renato fixing his Zeiss Super Ikonta on the sand and handling the thermometer, the exposure meter and the barometer, "the morning air is usually clearer and more transparent and brings a brighter light to the lens." "The afternoon has warmer colors and the sunset can give you shades that no other time of the day can offer." I attended countless discussions between the two brothers on the subject that was to be portrayed, on the position to choose for a shot, as well as the angles. Sometimes we would go home with nothing done because the two fussy photographers had believed that there were no conditions for the shot to fix the true soul of the landscape. More extemporaneous, animated and lively were the photos of the town that fixed moments of particular life, such as the Christmas lights in the center, a market day at the Boario Forum or exceptional situations such as the great snowfall of 1957 or the flood of 1966. I remember that on this occasion, after photographing the Carli square, which had literally become a lake in front of the town hall, we immediately returned to the shop and I was able to witness the development process of the sheets with the special developing solutions. It seemed to me that the images that surfaced highlighted both the sadness for the damage and devastation done by the water and the relief and joy that people felt for the narrow escape. For me it was like seeing Uncle Renato's thoughts and emotions surface and the developed film was the mirror of his soul.

Even today, I still live the places and people of the Altopiano through the lens of Uncle Renato, loaded with experienced emotions. After arriving from the hairpin bends of the Costo and taking the Canaglia valley beyond the old station of Campiello, I see the place where we used to hang out and wait for la Vacamora, the old train with the rising black plume of smoke that would arrive chugging and clattering. Now only thing that remains are the black and white postcards printed by the Bonomo brothers. And while I stop and get out of the car, I find another person who seems to look at the path where the rails have all but disappeared, with the same nostalgia that I feel for the scents, the noises, the coolness of the sparkling air of the forest that I felt as a boy, together with the excitement of seeing that locomotive pass tired but still working. It is Toio, the old ambulance driver from the Asiago hospital. He recognized me, nodding and said "Also you professor, are enjoying the panorama?" Then he proceeded to tell me about when my father had called him to take urgent patients to the hospital. He had established a bond with my father that seems to still exist and he speaks to me almost as if he were talking to him "because" he confesses to me, "when we see you in Asiago, we all see him, our old doctor."

And that is exactly how I live in the country today.

Five years ago, they gave me the honorary citizenship of this community, which does not lack sentimentality nor tenderness. They allowed me to be an Asiago doc for acquired merits. Perhaps many of these merits are those acquired by my father, but the villagers today greet me as one of them. They see in me a friend and a doctor who has never abandoned the roots of my youth. They know they can ask me, because they will receive listening and friendship. They enjoy giving me the more informal Italian "tu" (you) rather than "lei" (formal you), when they hear other important people give me the lei and they know that they can count on their closeness to me. They tell me about their old aunts or their elderly father and ask me advice, sometimes medical and sometimes just about life. With all of them I have maintained that unique relationship that can only be lived within a mountain community. I like when people stop to talk to me and tell me about my father or tell me about the old traditions of the woods and mountains. I like it when some lady tells my medical son about his grandfather Aldo would always leave some money on the cupboard for the poor instead of asking for a fee. I like to know that my son and I can adhere to my father's model as a doctor. I like it that the Asiaghesi are the ones that remind me of this. Their way of being friends makes me peaceful. It is as if they saw me inside and knew they were part of the important moments of my life. In turn, I keep these moments of friendship and simplicity as shots of an ideal camera that has a lens like that of Uncle Renato. Through it I can see my soul.

Epilogue

It is four o'clock in the afternoon on Christmas Eve and I'm sitting in the waiting room of a hospital. The heat from the radiator and the effects of jetlag returning from a seminar in the United States, brings sleepiness and my mind wanders to a Christmas Eve many years ago, when I was just beginning my medical career. I had been called urgently by the emergency room switchboard. I rushed in. "they brought us this 18-year-old American soldier" the doctor on duty told me. "He is back from the war front and seems to have ingested a great deal of drugs to kill himself." I looked at the soldier. He was little more than a boy. He had fear in his eyes. I asked him where he was from "Oklahoma City" he said grimly. I tell him, "I also know America. I have been there many times and I also went to your part where I ate the biggest hamburger of my life." He is silent and doesn't want to talk, but I insist. I have to keep him awake and understand what he has taken. "What's your name." "Peter." "What happened to you Peter?" "I felt so alone. It was Christmas Eve and I no longer wanted to live." I started talking to him in "New York slang" to tell him about my passion for the

Super Bowl, American hockey championships and other nonsense important for "us Americans." I try and make him feel that I too am a bit American and that he can feel at home with me. I explain to him that his kidneys are damaged and that I have to insert a catheter and do dialysis. I explain it to him in the same language and same terms as the American colleagues. He was trembling and I didn't know if it was from the poisoning or if he was just afraid. "Don't worry" I reassured him. "Stay calm and we'll spend a few hours in good company." He kept staring at me with wide eyes. I asked Rita to prepare the dialysis machine, we inserted the catheter and were ready to go. Blood rushed into the circuit as the pumps turned and cleaned the body of the killer poisons. Within a few hours, sitting by his side, I see life returning to Peter's veins. He is finally better, and I can also go home for Christmas Eve. I took off my lab coat and passed in front of the kitchen where the nurses were having coffee. I heard Rita tell the others about the particular filter that was applied to Peter, a prototype designed by me and made by some engineer friends. In the end, she exclaimed "This really saved our Doctor Ronco!"

Hearing my name woke me. Probably I had fallen asleep and was dreaming about my past. I stretched from the uncomfortable position that I had been in for nearly twenty minutes in the stiff chair. I couldn't fully grasp where I was. I knew I was in a hospital, because I heard again "This has really saved our Doctor Ronco." The nurse pronounced my name with great affection, but the voice wasn't that of Rita, and I understood that I wasn't in my hospital. I looked at the plaque on the door with the frosted glass that read "Hemodynamics Unit." At that moment, the door opened and Federico, my son, my playmate of the past, and now my colleague, wears the blue coat with the screen sealed to protect himself from radiation. He sees me and come towards me. "For the moment, I'm done. The patient emerged great. Let's go celebrate Christmas Eve Papa."

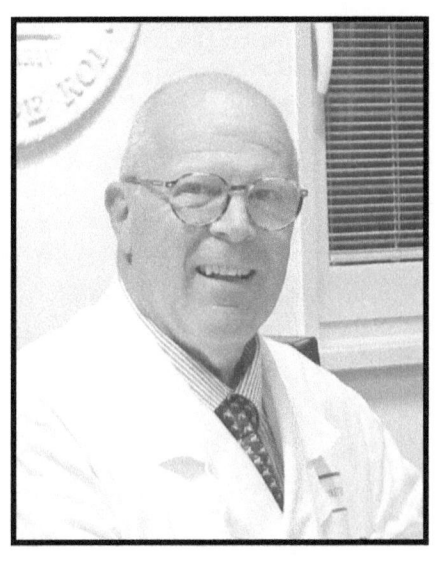

About the Author

Claudio Ronco, M.D. founded, and is the current Director of, the *International Renal Research Institute of Vicenza* (IRRIV) — a focal learning center of International young scientists, engineers and physicians with objectives of developing technology and cures for renal disease. Born in 1951, he grew up in Asiago, Italy, the son of the town doctor. He was previously director of the Beth Israel Renal Research Laboratories in New York, and teaches at both Padua and Bologna Universities. He is Professor of Medicine at the University of Virginia and at the Fudan and Jiaotong Universities in Shanghai.

He has published over a thousand scientific works and over eighty books which are used worldwide. Professor Ronco was nominated in 2014 as the John Hopkins University Top Scientist for Kidney Disease.

The Connectivist / Il Connettivista (First Edition) was first published in Italian in 2020.

www.ingramcontent.com/pod-product-compliance
Lightning Source LLC
Chambersburg PA
CBHW021425070526
44577CB00001B/62